WHY MILLIONS SURVIVE CANCER

WHY MILLIONS
SURVIVE CANCER

The Successes of Science

LAUREN PECORINO

OXFORD
UNIVERSITY PRESS

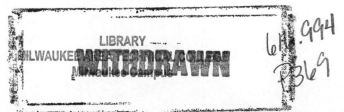

OXFORD

UNIVERSITY PRESS

Great Clarendon Street, Oxford OX2 6DP

Oxford University Press is a department of the University of Oxford.
It furthers the University's objective of excellence in research, scholarship,
and education by publishing worldwide in

Oxford New York

Auckland Cape Town Dar es Salaam Hong Kong Karachi
Kuala Lumpur Madrid Melbourne Mexico City Nairobi
New Delhi Shanghai Taipei Toronto

With offices in

Argentina Austria Brazil Chile Czech Republic France Greece
Guatemala Hungary Italy Japan Poland Portugal Singapore
South Korea Switzerland Thailand Turkey Ukraine Vietnam

Oxford is a registered trade mark of Oxford University Press
in the UK and in certain other countries

Published in the United States
by Oxford University Press Inc., New York

British Library Cataloguing in Publication Data

Data available

Library of Congress Cataloging in Publication Data

Data available

Typeset by SPI Publisher Services, Pondicherry, India
Printed in Great Britain
on acid-free paper by
Clays Ltd, St Ives plc

ISBN 978-0-19-958055-2

1 3 5 7 9 10 8 6 4 2

To my mother, Raffaela, who taught me compassion by example and my father, Joseph, who encourages the making of contributions to society.

CONTENTS

PREFACE

The idea for this book came from reading the feedback on Amazon.com about a textbook I had written on cancer biology. The feedback was posted by a cancer survivor who had been driven to reading a university textbook to learn more about the science of cancer. His determination to understand the molecular science of the disease, most likely without any previous specialized knowledge of the subject, was evident and it compelled me to write a book for the public. As a molecular biologist who greatly enjoys teaching a course in Cancer Biology and Therapeutics at the University of Greenwich, London, the above experience made me want to share the current knowledge of cancer biology with a wider audience. In describing the science behind the disease, two more themes became apparent.

Why Millions Survive Cancer: The Successes of Science is a book with three themes: the first is that over the last few decades we have built a far better scientific understanding of the disease and of the human body's remarkable defense against tumors; the second is that there is recent progress in our management of cancer and this is changing our view of the disease; and the last but most important is that evidence-based science informs us about lifestyle choices that reduce our risk of cancer and such changes in lifestyle save many lives.

The science is fascinating. Most topics about the mechanics of our body are of interest because they help define who we are. But the molecular world of how each individual cell works is another dimension that eludes most people in everyday life. Like a scuba diver immersed in the unfamiliar dimension of the ocean who marvels at the new surroundings, I hope that the reader becomes immersed in the molecular biology of our cells and finds an appreciation for this new world.

Statistics produced by international organizations are provided as evidence that there has been substantial recent progress against cancer. There can be no doubt that there is major progress: there are 28 *million* cancer survivors worldwide. This progress may be little known and was unexpected, even among cancer specialists.

Current lifestyle recommendations to prevent cancer and the experimental evidence that supports these recommendations are included as a platform for change. Advice on lifestyle changes can be found in many sources, but the most reliable are those backed by evidence. The evidence cited in this book has been published in peer-reviewed journals; that is, experts in the field are called upon to review each paper before it is published. Of course, this procedure is not foolproof, but it is one of the most reliable means currently available.

Each chapter opens with a quote from an expert in the field and gives a personal perspective about the progress against cancer reported in the chapter.

Statistical information is presented from original sources or in summary tables. Biological concepts are clearly explained and supported by easy-to-follow diagrams and published experimental data. Diagrams are a powerful tool for learning and the reader is asked to take a challenge and recall a specific diagram that is critical for fluent understanding of a central concept (see Chapter 5). Some images are provided as color plates.

Both a Bibliography and a Glossary are included at the end of the book. The Glossary defines unfamiliar words, highlighted in bold at first mention in the text, in a clear and concise manner for easy access. The Bibliography contains references found in the text and articles for interest as further reading, and includes primary research papers, easy-to-read reviews, and professional websites for the latest updates on national and international recommendations.

It is my hope that the readers of this book will learn something new, be entertained by the process of science and gain an appreciation of its efforts, and be able to guide others and themselves towards choosing a healthier lifestyle.

ACKNOWLEDGMENTS

First, I would like to express my thanks to Latha Menon, Commissioning Editor at Oxford University Press, for her belief in my original proposal. Thanks also to Emma Marchant, Assistant Commissioning Editor, and the production staff at Oxford University Press for their assistance, and to Nik Prowse, freelance copy-editor. With love, I thank my illustrator, my father Joseph Pecorino, for sharing his talents once again for the creation of many of the diagrams in the text. I am grateful to Marcus Gibson for his creative input, never-ending and kind support, regular press releases and news feeds, and the idea for the title of the book.

Kind appreciation is expressed for the precise and critical comments given by my official reviewers, especially Richard Grose (Institute of Cancer, Queen Mary's School of Medicine and Dentistry, UK).

Kind appreciation is also given for the willingness, time, and valuable comments from my unofficial reviewers who kindly read all or selected chapters: Alaisdair Stewart (Medway Hospital), Steven O'Grady, Charlie Pecorino, Sir Richard Peto (Oxford), John Schiller (National Cancer Institute), John Spencer (University of Greenwich), Tatiana Christides (University of Greenwich), and Heather Hampel (Ohio State University), and especially Lesley Walker (Cancer Research UK). World Cancer Research Fund International gave valuable advice relating to the chapter on nutrition.

I acknowledge all the scientists and doctors who dedicate their lives to cancer research and cancer patients. They are heroes. Special thanks to the scientists and experts who provided me with quotes for the opening of each chapter.

I am grateful to the University of Greenwich for providing me with years of opportunities to teach and develop my interest in cancer biology and I thank my Head of School, Martin Snowden, for his continual support of my writing projects. The School of Science, University of Greenwich, has provided me with financial support to attend the American Association for Cancer Research annual conferences. The information gained and the contacts made were important resources for this book. The Royal Society of Medicine, London hosted numerous lectures which contributed valuable information to this book, especially the innovation series hosted by Paul Summerfield.

Special thanks are expressed to David Lyden (Weill Medical College of Cornell University), Kirsty Beck (World Cancer Research Fund), Kelly Dobben-Annis (Cell Signaling Technology), and Tracy Walker and Fatima York (Siemens) for helping me to obtain electronic figures which add color and meaning to the words in the text. I would like to thank Marion Morra and my friend Marilyn Croucher for sharing some of their experiences with me. Thanks also to the support from Michael Caligiuri (Ohio State University).

I am grateful for the foundation of my scientific career set by my friends from the Strickland Laboratory and others from the State University of New York at Stony Brook during my PhD studies, and from the Brockes Laboratory at the Ludwig Institute for Cancer Research in London. I am especially grateful to the love and support that came from my family, especially Raffaela Pecorino and Teresa Rapillo, and from my friends.

LIST OF ILLUSTRATIONS
AND PLATES

ILLUSTRATIONS

PLATES

Plate 1 P53 becomes active in cells after UV treatment. Fluorescent reagents that bind to active P53 [phospho-P53 (Ser-15) (16G8) mouse monoclonal antibody (green)] were used in confocal immunofluorescent analysis of (A) untreated or (B) UV-treated cells. Actin filaments of the cells' cystoskeleton were labeled with Alexa Fluor 555 phalloidin (red) for contrast. Courtesy of Cell Signaling Technology, MA, USA. www.cellsignal.com.

Plate 2 Annual age-adjusted cancer death rates among males for selected cancers in the USA, 1930–2006. Note: the first ban on smoking in public buildings is indicated by the arrow. *US Mortality* Data, 1960 to 2006, US Mortality Volume 1930 to 1959. National Center for Health Statistics, Centers for Disease Control and Prevention. © Copyright 2010 American Cancer Society, with permission from John Wiley and Sons.

Plate 3 Estimated age-standardized mortality rate per 100,000 for cervix uteri, all ages. Ferlay J. et al., GLOBOCAN (2008) *Cancer Incidence and Mortality Worldwide: IARC CancerBase No. 10.* Lyon: International Agency for Research on Cancer, 2010.

Plate 4 Evidence of the premetastatic niche. Top row: bone marrow-derived cells form the premetastatic niche. Initiation: bone marrow-derived cells cluster in the lung before tumor cells arrive. Progression: migrating tumor cells adhere and grow specifically at these sites. Completion: blood vessel cells form vessels and are required for completion of the vascularized metastatic tumor. Green, bone marrow-derived cells; red, tumor cells; blue, nuclear staining, yellow, overlap of green and red; circular outline, a blood vessel within the metastatic tumor. Bottom row: a schematic of the formation of the premetastatic niche and metastatic process. Bone marrow-derived cells form clusters that initiate changes to the microenvironment that are necessary for future metastasis. For example, the non-cellular material called fibronectin is produced by fibroblast cells after bone marrow cells arrive. Adhesion and proliferation of tumor cells occur at these clusters. Blood vessel formation follows. Green, bone marrow-derived cells; T, tumor cell (red); FN, fibronectin (yellow); FB, fibroblasts (orange); TB, terminal bronchiole of the lung; BV, bronchiole vein of the lung.

1

INTRODUCTION
TO THE GOOD NEWS

There is no one universal target to attack in the war against cancer.
Instead there are many, possibly even hundreds. Despite this
complexity and the significant challenges that we face in curing
or preventing this disease, I have never been so confident that we
are now poised to take advantage of the wealth of discoveries that
cancer researchers have made over the last 25 years.

Joan Brugge, Chair, Department of Cell Biology, Harvard Medical School

Cancer is a disease that carries a lifetime risk of one in three.
Think about the neighbors on your street or the people in
your office and then think of the figure: one in three. In everyday
terms, cancer is pretty common, more common than most of us
care to admit. We all know someone who has had the disease. Cancer affects people of all nationalities and from all walks of life. No
one is exempt from the possibility of getting cancer.

Many people write books because they have a story to tell or a message to send. I am writing this book to send a message to as many
people as I can possibly reach. The message is meant to turn the 'one

in three' into something less common and to give those 'ones' hope. These aims may sound ambitious but the power of knowledge is bound to cause change. In my attempt to convey the message an unexpected story emerges. It is a true story, and it is remarkable. It is about the biology of our bodies that strives to protect us from cancer.

An extraordinary transformation has occurred in our perception, management, and treatment of cancer and this book is an evidence-based report on the good news about cancer. The news and messages in this book are supported by scientific data produced by the experts in the field.

One piece of good news is that now we find it acceptable to talk about cancer. The media talks about it, doctors talk about it, and even the people who have it, talk about it. Athletes such as Lance Armstrong, singers such as Kylie Minogue and Sheryl Crowe, and politicians such as Ted Kennedy have put a face on patients with cancer. These people have shown us that there is quality of life and hope after cancer. Real people also help to put a meaning behind statistics. Even small percentages of improvement in extending survival and quality of life equate to more time for active living for many people. *Stand Up to Cancer*, a celebrity-filled US national television fundraiser, sponsored by the American Association for Cancer Research, was a great occasion to raise awareness. Not only do well-known celebrities share their experiences of cancer, but our society gives celebrity status to cancer survivors who spread hope and positive attitudes in local communities. Cancer is a topic embedded in politics. Governmental policies from many countries include strategies for combating cancer.

Knowing about cancer on a personal level is important for everyone because of the statistics: one in three. It is the understanding and essence of biology that tells us what we should be doing. Individuals who know more about the disease may choose to make lifestyle changes to decrease their risk of cancer. Decreasing some risks of getting cancer is a matter of choice. The use of sunscreens and the cessation of smoking are two examples of how public awareness changes lifestyles and yields results. And I think people are becoming aware that they should know more about cancer. On one of my most recent cross-Atlantic flights my youthful neighbor remarked, in a matter-of-fact manner, that he had the feeling that he would get cancer one day. His concern was not immediate, and rightly so. Generally cancer risk increases with age.

For most cancers, development is a multi-step process that involves the accumulation of small changes to our cells over time, but it is worthy to note that recent evidence suggests that in some cases, cancer can develop from a single cellular castrophe that results in massive chromosomal damage and large numbers of mutations (Stephens et al., 2011). The words of the young man sitting next to me on the plane are a testimony to progress, showing that some people truly understand their own personal risk and feel free to broach the subject in a casual setting.

Some people have stated that they feel that cancer is more common now than it has been historically. There are several reasons that one may feel like this. First, many diseases and infections that once killed people at an early age have been eliminated or at least controlled. Smallpox, tuberculosis, and childhood diseases are examples. As a result of better medicine and improved quality of life, people are living longer. Sixty is the new 40. So, in the last century, fewer people lived long enough to develop cancer. Another reason that cancer may appear to be more common today is that a few generations ago cancer was not discussed. Doctors would call a tumor a cyst or avoid the word 'cancer' and call it 'the big C' instead. The good news is that cancer **incidence rates** (the number of new cases per population in a given period) have been decreasing over recent years in the USA, as reported in Cancer Statistics, 2010 (Jemal et al., 2010a). One factor that contributes to this good news and underlies the accelerated decrease in colorectal cancer incidence rates from 1998 to 2006 in the USA is screening, which can detect and remove precancerous polyps. Other factors that underlie this good news of decreasing incidence rates are revealed in later chapters.

The importance of public awareness cannot be over-emphasized. A survey sponsored by the Union for International Cancer Control (UICC), based on 40,000 people in 39 countries, strongly suggests that people in both developed and developing countries have misunderstandings about what causes cancer (Machlin et al., 2009). The survey found, for example, that 25% of people who drink alcohol frequently and also use tobacco daily believe that smoking cigarettes does not increase the risk of cancer. An educated population can make better and informed choices and help influence policy. The policy of banning smoking in public places caused a social activity to become antisocial, and led to obvious health benefits which we will examine in Chapter 4. The fact that we can make lifestyle changes to decrease cancer risk needs to be emphasized. Actually, it needs to be screamed from the highest mountain!

Another piece of good news is that information about cancer is accessible and can easily be shared. The internet is making a vast amount of information available to all. We have access to official, unofficial, and personal information. But, along with this great supply of information, there is a need for the public to be educated to understand the information and, more importantly, how to be critical of the source and the content of the information. In a capitalistic world we have become vigilant consumers, learning to read the fine print on advertisements to avoid the latest scam. We have learned that you don't get something for nothing. Similarly we must learn to scrutinize information about cancer. Headlines claiming that there is a cure for all cancers obtained from a pit of a rare tropical fruit should be read with caution. In the USA it is illegal to offer a cure for cancer or to offer advice on treatment outside of the medical profession under the Cancer Act of 1939. This doesn't mean that people do not try to make their fortunes by such a route. People advertising cancer cures on the internet have been convicted in recent years. Cancer is a very complex disease and it is extremely unlikely that there will be one magic bullet to cure all cases. The complexity of the biology of the disease should become apparent in the pages ahead. Having a glimpse at the complexity should help to soothe the anger that is sometimes expressed by patients who are 'mad as hell' as they exclaim, 'If we can put a man on the moon why can't we cure cancer?' Simply, the answer is: 'going to the moon is much easier'.

The testing of new drugs must be carried out in stages. Knowledge about the genetics or physiology of a cancer identifies a target and chemicals that can attack the target are identified/produced and tested. The usual route is that a potential drug demonstrates an effect on a cancer cell line (cancer cells grown in the laboratory) or in an animal tumor model before being tested in humans in clinical trials. Phase I clinical trials examine drug dose and drug safety using a small number (20–80) of healthy volunteers or patients. Phase II clinical trials test how well the drug works in a larger group (100–300) of people. Phase III studies are large-scale studies (1000–3000 people) that further examine drug efficiency, side-effects, and effectiveness compared to currently used treatments. Only about 16% of drugs tested are successful in moving from Phase I to approval (DiMasi et al., 2010). This process is long and expensive but it strives to ensure safety for the public. The individuals who volunteer to enter trials are heroes because they may be sacrificing their health for the good of future generations.

The *best* news is that we are living in an age where we are finally witnessing progress being made in the war against cancer. This was a war declared by the US President, Richard Nixon, in his State of the Union address in 1971. Soon after, the National Cancer Act enabled the expansion and creation of Comprehensive Cancer Centers in the USA. Making headway against the enemy of cancer was not an easy task, even for a world superpower. For so many years it has felt like a losing battle. But the tides are changing, and changing rapidly.

Here are two striking examples of recent good news about cancer. The most impressive is a report that examined trends in death rates, a robust measure of progress against cancer, from scientists at the American Cancer Society (Jemal et al., 2010b). Trends in death rates reflect changes in prevention, diagnosis, and treatment. The study used US national data and computer software to standardize data from 1970 through 2006. The results are clear and significant (Figure 1): there is progress in reducing cancer death rates measured against rates of both 1970 and 1990 (the year when all-cancer death rates peaked). The death rate for men has shown a

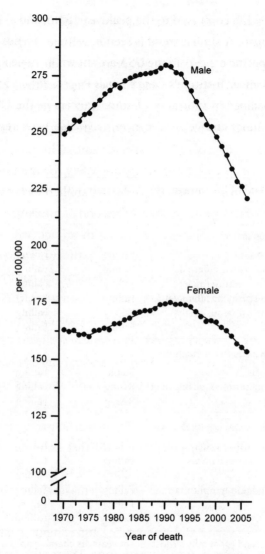

FIG 1 Trends in age-standardized death rates for all cancers combined by sex, 1970–2006. Dots represent observed rates and solid lines fitted rates.

decrease of 21% compared to the peak year, 1990, and a decline of 11% from 1970. A similar trend is seen in women. Trends in death rates for specific cancers in the USA are shown in Table 1 from the National Cancer Institute's *Cancer Trends Progress Report 2009/2010 Update*. Declines in mortality of some cancers in the USA, such as breast, lung, and cervical cancer, have also been reported in

Measure: end of life (mortality)	Recent trend*	Desired direction
All cancers	Falling	Falling
Most common cancers		
• Female breast	Falling	Falling
• Colon and rectum (female)	Falling	Falling
• Colon and rectum (male)	Falling	Falling
• Lung and bronchus (female)	Falling	Falling
• Lung and bronchus (male)	Falling	Falling
• Prostate	Falling	Falling
Cancers with increasing mortality rate		
• Esophagus	Stable	Falling
• Liver and intrahepatic bile duct	Rising	Falling
• Pancreas	Rising	Falling
Cancers with decreasing mortality rate		
• Brain and other system	Falling	Falling
• Kidney and renal pelvis	Falling	Falling
• Myeloma	Falling	Falling
• Non-Hodgkin lymphoma	Falling	Falling
• Ovary	Falling	Falling
• Stomach	Falling	Falling

*Summary trend (generally 5 most recent years) as characterized by the average annual percent change (AAPC).

Table 1. Trends in mortality in the USA for specific cancers. From National Cancer Institute (2010) *Cancer Trends Progress Report – 2009/2010 Update*. April 2010. http://progressreport.cancer.gov/trends-glance.asp.

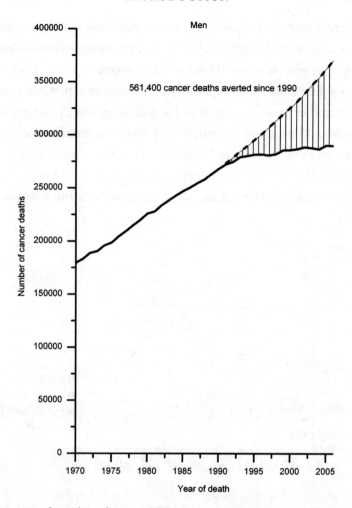

FIG 2 Total number of cancer deaths (in men) averted due to reduction in cancer death rates since 1990. Solid lines represent the observed number of cancer deaths and dashed lines expected cancer deaths. Expected cancer deaths are based on extrapolation of the peak rates in men (1990) to 2006.

several European countries, Australia, and Canada. The decrease is the result of decreasing tobacco use, increased screening, and improvements in treatment for specific cancers.

An illustration of the meaning of this decrease in death rates in terms of years of potential life gained in men is shown in Figure 2. Researchers compared death rates expected had the peak rates remained unchanged (dashed line) to the actual number of cancer deaths (solid line). This comparison shows that 561,400 cancer deaths have been averted since 1990. Note these data are

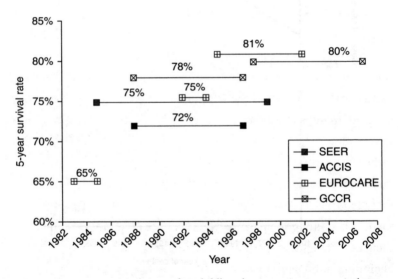

FIG 3 Five-year survival rates for childhood cancer (0–14 years) drawn from different data sources reporting different time periods. *Sources*: ACCIS (1988–1997), EUROCARE (1983–1985, 1992–1994, 1995–2002), GCCR (1988–1997, 1998–2007), SEER (1985–1999) (ACCIS, European Automated Childhood Cancer Information System; SEER, US-Surveillance, Epidemiology and End Results; GCCR, German Childhood Cancer Registry).

only for men in the USA. The number or cancer deaths averted for men and women, worldwide, is over a million.

Another example of the recent good news about cancer is the results from the analysis of the most valid European data set existing at present for childhood cancers (Kaatsch, 2010). In developed countries, cancer is the second most common cause of death in childhood. One can see from the data in Figure 3 that the five-year survival rates for childhood cancer have increased for the more recent time periods. The change from 65% for the period 1982–1985 to 81% for more recent years is personally comforting to see because I lost a childhood friend to leukemia in 1980. Similar improvements are seen in the USA.

Overall, the good news about cancer is that there is progress. It is estimated that there are 28 *million* cancer survivors worldwide (with about 12 million in the USA alone). Treatments are becoming gentler and more effective. Many newly developed drugs have fewer side-effects and can be administered in the form of a pill rather than intravenous administration, giving patients a better quality of life. Better response rates are occurring for treatments that are targeted against genetic characteristics of a tumor. Treatment is becoming increasingly personalized to an individual and their cancer. This progress is fairly recent and it just may be the beginning of the end.

2

WHAT IS CANCER?

If we wish to learn more about cancer, we must
now concentrate on the cellular genome.

Renato Dulbecco, Nobel Laureate, from Science *(Dulbecco, 1986)*

What is cancer? Before tackling that question, let's consider how cancer is perceived by looking at some personal viewpoints. A project aimed at addressing information needs of teenage cancer patients, called 'What colour is my cancer?' based at St James's University Hospital, Leeds, UK, reported that many teenagers with cancer perceived it as evil aliens that took over their body. Their perception changed after being given the chance to view their own cancer through a microscope. Descriptions of cancer by adults are similar. When asking a friend who had been diagnosed with breast cancer to define cancer in her own words she said '[it is a] nasty critter a bit like a maggot in an apple. If you leave it, the maggot will eventually destroy the fruit. Cut it out and the fruit lasts longer.' When Charlotte met her lifelong partner, it was love at first sight. Although there was a slight language barrier between his Polish and her English, they communicated well. Even when he said that his dad had been eaten by a crab, she understood that his father had died of cancer.

Cancer is commonly perceived as something foreign that takes over (and eats) your body. This perception is powerful but has some major flaws. Changing this widespread view of cancer may have important implications for its prevention.

A useful analogy for cancer involves thinking about the human body as a car. Car trouble is usually due to wear and tear. How it is driven and maintained has a large effect on a car's 'health'. Most car owners know that dirty or diluted fuel can damage an engine; thus the quality of fuel input is a prime importance in the care of a car. The risk of getting cancer depends on lifestyle and maintenance. Similar to putting high-quality fuel into a car, consuming high-quality fuel in the form of a healthy diet and trying to avoid harmful substances, like cigarette smoke, is part of good maintenance. The quality of a car's parts also plays a hand. Cancer is also dependent on the quality of our parts, which is dictated by our genes. And, the older the car the more likely it is to have car trouble. The older we are, the greater the risk of cancer. This is because, in most cases, cancer is a multi-step process that involves the accumulation of damage over time. Understanding cancer allows us to understand our individual risk of getting cancer, remembering that for most of the population this is one in three.

This chapter will focus on answering the question, 'what is cancer?' First let's examine cancer compared to other diseases. Anemia is a disease of the blood, Alzheimer's disease is a disease of the brain, and blindness is a disease of the eyes. Cancer can be found in many different organs. In fact, cancer is not one disease but it is a *set* of diseases. There are many different types of cancer that are named by the organ where it first appears: skin cancer, lung cancer, liver cancer, brain cancer, etc. Each type of cancer is caused by different agents. For example, ultraviolet radiation from the sun causes skin cancer but not lung cancer. Smoking causes lung cancer but not skin cancer. Treatment of each type of cancer may be different. Procedures for removing a brain tumor are a lot more complex than for removing some skin cancers.

Cancer has two main characteristics: it is characterized by abnormal cell growth and the ability to spread to other parts of the body (metastasis). Let's look at these characteristics a little more closely. A wart, a pimple, and a benign tumor are examples of abnormal cell growth but none of these are cancer. In contrast, a malignant tumor which displays both abnormal cell growth *and* the ability to spread throughout the body is evidence of cancer. Both of these characteristics, and not just one alone, are needed to define cancer.

To understand why the disease occurs in different organs, a discussion of the disease at its most basic core is needed. Cancer occurs because of alterations that lead to permanent changes (**mutations**) of specific **genes**. The reason that there are so many types of cancer is that genes are found in every type of cell in the body and so every cell can be a candidate for the origin of cancer.

GENES, THE TARGET OF CANCER

One of the most rewarding aspects of studying the biology of cancer for so many years is that you really begin to appreciate the remarkable precision and efficiency of the workings of a normal healthy cell. A cell carries out many of the activities of the whole individual. A cell requires nutrients and oxygen, carries out work, communicates with other cells, reproduces, responds to stress, etc. The instructions needed for cells to function are contained in our genes and are written using only four letters: A, G, C, and T. The letters stand for small chemical molecules called adenine, guanine, cytosine, and thymine, respectively. These four molecules are called bases. The linear order of these bases along the length of a chromosome makes up genes, like letters make up words. Genes provide instructions to make all the products (proteins) needed to make the body function. In general, one gene codes for one protein product. Some genes code for proteins that help different cells communicate with each other, some for products that make up what we look like (skin pigment, eye color, material for curly or straight hair), and others code for proteins that carry out biochemical reactions such as those involved in digestion that allow us to get energy from food. The Human Genome Project, a herculean effort to read all of the genes in human cells, the **genome**, has revealed that humans have about 25,000 genes.

Genes are made of deoxyribonucleic acid, or **DNA**. The molecular structure of DNA, elucidated by the famous duo James Watson and Francis Crick, is remarkable in its simplistic nature and its function. It acts as a digital storage device and execution of the information defines life. Two strands of DNA wrap around each other to form a twisted ladder or double helix. Pairs of the bases A, G, C, and T mentioned above make up the rungs of the ladder. The pairing occurs in a particular way: C always pairs with G (and vice versa); A always pairs with T (and vice versa). This specific base-pairing rule allows the sequence of any gene to be easily copied:

by knowing the sequence of one strand, a matching strand can be made.

Before a cell divides the DNA must be precisely replicated so that each daughter cell receives a complete set of genes. The two strands of the double helix separate. The precise pairing rules allow each of the strands to act as a template for the production of a new strand of DNA (Figure 4). During the process of mitosis, the duplicated chromosomes are split evenly into two daughter cells. Each daughter cell then contains a complete copy of genes.

Maintaining the integrity of the DNA during cell growth (the process of making more cells) is important. Remember that DNA codes for instructions that are translated to carry out all functions necessary for life; loss or change of DNA can have severe consequences.

The link between the biology of genes and cancer becomes clear as one examines what causes cancer. Many agents that cause cancer, called **carcinogens**, are commonly known: smoking, ultraviolet rays from the sun, radiation, and some chemicals. Most carcinogens target genes and ultimately cause mutations in the DNA sequence. Mutations may be the substitution of one base (ATGC) for another or may involve removal or addition of bases. The consequence of a mutation may be compared to errors in a musical score. The change of one note for another may sound awkward and the addition of a note or the removal of a note may alter the whole tempo of a song. Gene mutations may result in the production of an altered protein. Altered proteins may alter cell function. If the mutations fall within genes whose products are involved in regulating the cell numbers in the body (e.g. growth, cell death, or cell specialization) they may produce faulty proteins that lead

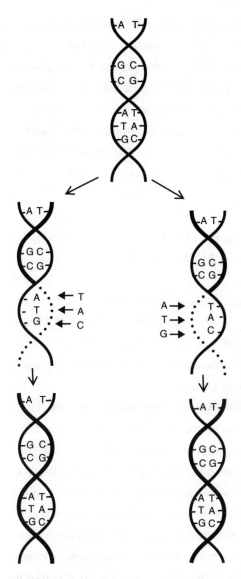

FIG 4 DNA replication. The two strands of DNA separate. Each strand can act as a template for the making of a new second strand using the specific base-pairing rule: C pairs with G (and vice versa) and A pairs with T (and vice versa). This process is precise and helps to maintain the integrity of the DNA sequence during cell division. Thick black lines represent the newly synthesized DNA strand.

to abnormal cell growth. An altered gene that produces a protein product that contributes to cancer is called an **oncogene**. **Tumor suppressor genes**, whose product is normally involved in blocking tumor formation, are another type of gene involved in cancer development. Mutations in tumor suppressor genes lead to nonfunctional tumor blockers and eliminate a natural defense against tumors. In fact, it is thought that it is not just one mutation, but an accumulation of mutations in different genes of a target cell, that leads to cancer.

YOU CAN'T (FULLY) BLAME GETTING CANCER ON YOUR MOM OR DAD

Mutations are the underlying cause of both cancer and inherited disease. A major difference between an inherited disease and cancer is *which genes* the mutations affect and whether the causative mutations occur in the sex cells (also known as germ cells: egg or sperm) or body cells (somatic cells).

Cancer is characterized by mutations in genes whose products affect net cell numbers, since cancer is a disease characterized by abnormal growth. Cell growth, cell suicide, and cell specialization are three processes that contribute to maintaining the net cell numbers in an individual. Cell growth produces more cells, cell suicide results in fewer cells, and when a cell becomes specialized it does not divide or die for a specific period of time. Let's examine a simple model, shown in Figure 5, to see how changes in these processes may give rise to abnormal cell numbers. If four cells of the nine cells shown in Figure 5a divide (÷), four commit cell suicide (X), and one cell becomes specialized (S) so that it

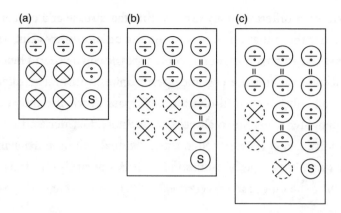

FIG 5 A simple model of processes that affect cell numbers. Cell division (÷), cell suicide (X), and cell specialization (S). Dashed outlines illustrate dead cells.

will neither divide nor die, the cell number will remain the same (Figure 5b). However, if cell suicide is blocked in one cell and this cell divides instead, the total number of cells will increase to 11 (Figure 5c). Similarly, if cell specialization is blocked in a cell and this cell divides instead (as is the case for leukemias), the number of cells will also increase. Therefore mutations in genes that affect the processes of growth, cell suicide, or specialization can alter cell numbers and contribute to the development of a tumor.

Take, on the other hand, patients with the inherited disease sickle cell anemia. They carry a mutation in the hemoglobin gene and as a consequence hemoglobin protein has an altered structure and function, giving rise to sickle-shape cells. A mutation in the hemoglobin gene does not give rise to cancer because hemoglobin does not have any functions that affect net cell growth.

Another difference between an inherited disease and cancer is whether the mutation occurs in the sex cells or body cells. The sickle cell anemia mutation is present in the egg or sperm before conception. After the egg and sperm unite to form a fertilized egg, all subsequent cell divisions will pass down the mutation to daughter cells. Since all cells in an individual descend from the fertilized egg, every cell in the individual will have the sickle cell gene. This type of mutation is called a **germline mutation** because the mutation was carried by the germ cells (either egg or sperm).

The mutational events that lead to cancer occur in cells of an individual during their lifetime. Cancer is said to be a genetic disease at the cellular level. The phrase 'at the cellular level' in this statement is important and distinguishes cancer from inherited diseases. In a cancer patient, the mutations originate in one single body (somatic) cell of an individual due to the exposure of carcinogens, and only descendent cells of the affected cell will carry the mutation. It is these descendent cells that form a tumor. This type of mutation is called a **somatic mutation** and, unlike a germline mutation, is not present in every cell of the body. These mutations are hardly ever passed down to offspring because the mutations are in somatic (body) cells in a specific location (e.g. a lung cell) and are not within sex cells (egg or sperm) that contribute to the formation of a new individual. So cancer is only very rarely inherited.

But, there are inherited cancer syndromes that may be passed down from generation to generation and affected individuals in these families have an increased risk of developing cancer. Below are a few examples. About 5–10% of all breast cancers are due to a hereditary syndrome whereby individuals who carry a specific germline mutation have an increased risk of developing breast cancer. Every cell of these individuals carries a mutation in one of two copies of a specific tumor suppressor gene. Inherited mutations in the *BRCA1* and *BRCA2* genes give patients an increased risk of breast cancer and ovarian cancer. The protein product of these genes plays a role in DNA repair, so acquiring a mutation in the second *BRCA1/2* genes can lead to a faulty DNA-repair system in cells. Such cells are susceptible to accumulating mutations, one of the underlying mechanisms for cancer development. These patients have a 'head-start' in a race that no one wants to win. Today we have the technology to test for *BRCA1/2* gene mutations. Results from such tests give us information that equips us for making better lifestyle choices, such as frequent breast cancer screening (discussed in Chapter 9).

Here is a case study that illustrates a family that is marked by a *BRCA* mutation. A mother of three is diagnosed with advanced-stage breast cancer. After receiving surgery and conventional chemotherapy she dies at the age of 45. Ten years later, one of her three daughters is diagnosed with early-stage breast cancer as a result of the national breast screening program. She receives a newly approved drug and has been disease-free for more than five years. The occurrence of breast cancer in two successive generations hinted that *BRCA1/2* gene mutations may exist in the family. The remaining two sisters were screened for *BRCA1/2* mutations. One sister is normal and therefore her risk of getting breast cancer is the same as the general population. The other sister carries the suspected mutation and, due to her increased risk of developing breast cancer, will be monitored closely and frequently. She has rejected the option of prophylactic surgery (removal of healthy breasts and/or ovaries as a means of removing 'at-risk' tissue) because even this radical approach is not a 100% guarantee for remaining cancer-free.

Another hereditary syndrome that results in an increased risk of cancer is familial adenomatous polyposis (FAP). Patients with this syndrome inherit a mutation in the *APC* gene. The product of this gene plays a role in regulating the growth of the stem cells of the colon, a tissue which, like the skin, regenerates itself regularly. Patients with this syndrome develop many polyps, precancerous legions that can go on to develop into cancer. It takes a second mutation to completely inactivate the two copies of the *APC* gene and to initiate colon cancer. Again, the patient has a head-start in the race to cancer.

Inborn metabolic disorders may also increase an individual's risk of cancer. An example can be easily illustrated by the disorder albinism. A person with albinism, an albino, is unable to produce the pigment called melanin. Albinos are striking against the normal population because they lack pigment in their skin, hair, and eyes. Since melanin provides some protection against the sun's ultraviolet rays, albinos have an increased risk of skin cancer.

So, the take-home message is most carcinogens are mutagens that target genes in somatic (body) cells of an individual over their lifetime. Mutations cause the production of faulty proteins that can lead to abnormal cell growth and ultimately cancer. Cancer is only rarely inherited but specific inherited germline mutations give those affected a head-start and increase the risk of getting cancer.

YOUR LIFESTYLE, AND CANCER

Lifestyle factors will influence your exposure to different carcinogens and play a role in cancer risk. The study of cancer, in different geographical locations, is enlightening because it shows that environment and lifestyle play a role in cancer. The Globocan 2008 website (accessed on http://globocan.iarc.fr/) is a useful and fascinating collection of data that allows you to choose a country from anywhere in the world and view cancer profiles of the population. For instance, the leading new cases of cancer in the USA for males are prostate, lung, and colon. The leading new cases of cancer in Ethiopia for males are Kaposi sarcoma, esophageal cencer, and non-Hodgkin lymphoma. Lung cancer does not appear on the Madagascar list because smoking is not common. Other countries such as Korea and Japan show a high number of new cases of stomach cancer. Studies of immigrants and the adoption of new diets suggest diet is a risk factor for stomach cancer. The mechanisms of how different carcinogens cause different cancers will be discussed in later chapters.

CHANCE

Chance is also part of the cancer story. To illustrate the risk of getting a cancer-causing mutation, picture a tremendous wall that can display all of your 3.4 billion base-pair sequence on a wall; yes, that's 3.4 billion As, Gs, Cs, and Ts. You are given a bucket full of darts each labeled with one base, A, G, T, or C. If you hit a base, it will change to the base on the dart. Steady, aim, and fire. Some of your darts may not hit the wall. Some direct hits may not cause a change in the sequence at all because, for example, you may hit an A in the sequence with a dart labeled with an A. Furthermore, only changes in about 290 genes of the 25,000 genes in the human genome may give rise to cancer. So far, the chances may seem slim. Now think that each cell of your body has such a dart board. It is estimated that you have between 50 and 100 trillion cells in your body! One can easily see how risk increases with this number of cells. Of course, this is a simplistic view and biology is more complicated. Later in the book we will examine how our body protects itself from mutations and how we can help by eating a healthy diet and being physically active. One lesson from the analogy is to try to decrease the number of darts in your bucket: avoid the carcinogens that you can.

UNDERSTANDING INFLUENCES TREATMENT

The observation that cancer is characterized by abnormal growth gave doctors a handle on how cancer could be treated. First, the abnormal growth, or tumor, is removed by surgery. Radiation is often given afterwards to kill any remaining cells that surgery did not remove and finally chemotherapy is given to attack cells that may have escaped from the original site and may be spreading to other sites in the body. These conventional cancer treatments save or at least prolong many lives. But, still the strategies are crude.

Cancer treatments are evolving over time, just like weapons of war have evolved over the ages. Early on weapons included large catapults which had poor aim and gave rise to extensive damage around the target. Similarly, surgery does not allow perfect aim; one can imagine that it is not easy to surgically remove *all* of the cells of a tumor with a scalpel. And we are all aware of the severe side-effects of chemotherapy. Chemotherapy is not selective against tumor cells; it also kills healthy, rapidly dividing cells such as hair follicles, intestinal cells, and blood cells. The common side-effects of hair loss, ulcers, and anemia, respectively, leave the patient feeling unwell. Both are brute-force attempts to kill the enemy/ cancer and produce damage in surrounding areas. But the future is brighter because we have entered a new age of targeted cancer therapies. Drugs are being designed to interfere with specific gene products that are known to be causative factors in a particular type of cancer. As we learn about the genes and gene products involved in cancer initiation and progression, we will be able to build a larger and more focused arsenal against the disease.

THE GOOD NEWS

As a result of our scientific understanding, a new perception of cancer is taking hold: our fate with regards to cancer is determined by our personal maintenance of health in our chosen lifestyle, by the hand of cards we have been dealt in terms of our genes, and by chance. Soon technology will allow us to read our individual hand of genes and we will have to learn how best to use this new information. Thoughts of cancer being caused by invading foreign aliens should be discarded and replaced by a scientific understanding and the realization that we have some control in determining our own individual risk of cancer.

Good news is that, over the years, improvements have been seen in all three modes of conventional treatment: surgery, radiation, and chemotherapy. Advances in instrumentation, robotics, and imaging have led to more precise and less invasive surgical procedures. In a study reported in *The Lancet* a refined technique of rectal cancer surgery, pioneered by the British surgeon Richard Heald, has been shown to halve the rate of recurrence (Martling et al., 2000). Also, 'dose-dense' chemotherapy schedules, which involve receiving treatment every 2 weeks instead of every 3 weeks, have been shown in clinical trials led by Larry Norton at Memorial Sloan-Kettering Cancer Center in New York to lower breast cancer recurrence by 26% over three years. This modification has become common practice for certain breast cancer patients at high risk of relapse. Patient-care drugs, such as Aranesp and Neulasta produced by the biotechnology company giant Amgen, have been developed to help alleviate side-effects of chemotherapy (anemia and low white-blood-cell count, respectively).

3

CARCINOGENS: HOW THEY
WORK AND OUR DEFENSE
AGAINST THEM

With an increasing identification of infectious agents being essential
components in the development of some widespread human
cancers, cancer prevention of these types of cancers
becomes more and more a realistic development.

*Harald zur Hausen, Nobel Laureate, 2008. German Cancer
Research Center, Heidelberg, Germany*

What causes cancer? The answer to the question is: carcinogens are agents that cause cancer. Known carcinogens
include tobacco smoke, radiation, certain chemicals, infectious
agents, and natural products. Carcinogens alter the structure of
DNA in particular cells, and these alterations lead to DNA damage.
Unrepaired DNA damage can lead to a permanent change in the
base sequence of DNA (mutation). Mutations include base substi-
tutions (one base is replaced with another), insertions (the addition
of a base), and deletions (loss of a base) (Figure 6). Mutations also
include chromosomal translocations where chromosomes break
and rejoin with a different chromosome. Mutations in genes

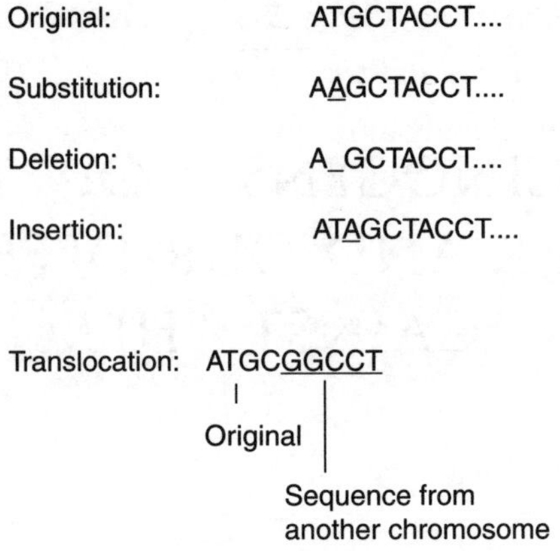

Original:	ATGCTACCT....
Substitution:	AAGCTACCT....
Deletion:	A_GCTACCT....
Insertion:	ATAGCTACCT....

Translocation: ATGCGGCCT
              |
         Original

                 Sequence from
                 another chromosome

FIG 6 Types of mutations, permanent changes to the base sequence of DNA. Mutations are underlined.

involved in cell growth, cell differentiation, or cell suicide, are passed down to daughter cells to initiate the formation of a tumor, as discussed in the previous chapter.

It may be comforting to know that we have efficient 'built-in' defense systems against carcinogens, including the ability of cells to repair DNA damage. But, like most systems, an overload to the system or a weakness can cause the system to give way. Exposure to carcinogens over long periods of time allows for an accumulation of damage. That's why cancer is generally a disease of aging: cancer development requires time.

This chapter explains *how* different types of carcinogens cause mutations. Such information strengthens our understanding of why something is potentially harmful. This knowledge can greatly influence individual lifestyle choices. It is impossible to escape from all known carcinogens, but better awareness may lead us to avoid exposure to certain carcinogens that we can control. The media is constantly reporting 'this' and 'that' causes cancer, sometimes with strong evidence and sometimes without it. There are several official sites that classify human carcinogens including the International Agency for Research on Cancer (IARC) and the US National Toxicology Program's Report of Carcinogens. Modern society has a good record for unknowingly increasing our exposure to carcinogens and so what is hailed as progress needs constant re-evaluation with respect to carcinogenic effects. Pesticides, fertilizers, food additives, and medical treatments have fallen under this guise. The mechanism of the most avoidable carcinogen, cigarette smoke, will be discussed in the next chapter. Radiation, chemicals, estrogen, and infectious agents are discussed below.

RADIATION

Radiation is energy. Electromagnetic radiation is a range of naturally occurring radiation ranging from low-energy types such as infrared, to high-energy types such as X-rays. Two types of radiation cause cancer: ultraviolet (UV) radiation and ionizing radiation. Both of these types of radiation have higher energy compared to radiowaves, infrared, and visible light.

UV radiation is a form of energy from the sun. Since UV does not penetrate the body more deeply than the skin, it is a carcinogen that is specific to skin. UV causes a type of DNA damage that is not observed with other carcinogens. The most common type of damage is called a pyrimidine dimer (a 'pyrimidine' is a C or T of the genetic code) caused by UVB (wavelength 290–320 nanometers): two Cs, or two Ts, or a C and a T, that lie next to each other in the DNA sequence chemically bond together to

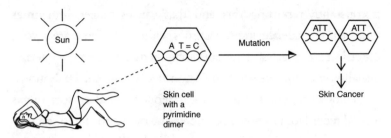

FIG 7 How does UV radiation cause skin cancer? UV radiation causes abnormal links between certain DNA bases to create pyrimidine dimers. Pyrimidine dimers can lead to mutations and eventually skin cancer.

form a dimer (two together) (Figure 7). This causes a bend in the DNA helix and as a result the DNA is misread by the enzyme that copies DNA during cell reproduction. The polymerase inserts an 'A' when reading a pyrimidine dimer, and this gives rise to a substitution mutation (a 'T' replaces a 'C') during the next round of DNA replication.

The mutation of one particular gene, called *p53*, is important for the initiation of skin cancer and also for other types of cancer. It is a tumor suppressor gene whose loss of function contributes to cancer. In healthy cells, the product of this gene, P53, is crucial for blocking tumor formation and plays an important role in the defense against skin cancer. The P53 product becomes active after UV exposure. This can be 'seen' in cells using fluorescent reagents that recognize active P53 (Plate 1). Staying in the sun too long early in the summer season often leads to the 'peeling' of our skin. This peeling is dying skin cells that have been ordered by P53 to commit cell suicide in response to extensive DNA damage. It is best for the individual to lose these damaged skin cells and prevent the risk of skin cancer. When the *p53* gene is itself damaged, its product cannot function properly and skin cells with extensive DNA damage from the sun remain rather than die. These cells may contribute to the initiation of skin cancer.

So, is a tanning salon a safer place to get a tan? The answer is *no*. Studies have shown that short-term visits to the tanning salon (as short as 10 sessions in 2 weeks) result in the same type of DNA damage as described above that contributes to the development of skin cancer.

The second type of radiation that causes cancer is ionizing radiation. Ionizing radiation, including X-rays, is a high-energy type of radiation that can displace an electron from a molecule. The molecule becomes charged, creating an **ion**. Hence ionizing radiation causes the formation of ions. Ionizing radiation can cause mutations directly by ionizing DNA. It can also damage DNA indirectly by interacting with water, the most abundant substance in living things, to create highly reactive oxygen molecules called **reactive oxygen species** (or ROS). The reactive oxygen species can oxidize DNA bases. Because both ionized and oxidized DNA bases 'appear different' they may be misread during replication and this can lead to mutations and ultimately cancer.

People receive varying amounts of ionizing radiation depending on the altitude and location of where they live, how many flights they take, or how many X-rays they have. (Note: exposure to radon gas from the earth will be discussed in the next chapter.) Ionizing radiation from outer space (cosmic radiation) continually bombards the earth. People who live in high altitudes such as Denver, Colorado, in the USA are exposed to more cosmic radiation than people who live at lower altitudes, such as Chicago. This is because people are closer to outer space in Denver compared to Chicago and there is less atmosphere to shield them. The exposure for a US cross-country flight in a commercial airplane (2–5 millirem) is less than one half of the exposure of a chest X-ray. Several studies of the effects of radiation during commercial flights to flight crew have been published: some show no increased risk but other studies show an increase of specific cancers. For example, one study published in *The Lancet* in 1999 showed that male cockpit crew members in jets flying more than 5000 hours have a significantly increased frequency of acute myeloid leukemia (Gundestrup and Storm, 1999). Ionizing radiation can cause chromosomal breaks that lead to chromosomal translocations. Chromosomal translocations are common in leukemia. Victims of the atomic bombs that hit Japan during World War II received very high doses of ionizing radiation. A long-term and comprehensive study of 80,000 atomic bomb survivors, called the Life Span Study, is revealing important information about radiation exposure and helps guide recommendations for radiation limits. The first and most frequent cancer to be associated with atomic-bomb radiation exposure was leukemia but excess risks of most cancer types have been observed; those exposed as children carry the highest risk of radiation-induced cancer (Preston et al., 2003; Little, 2009). The US National Council on Radiation Protection and Measurements (NCRP) and the International Commission on Radiological Protection recommends an annual radiation dose limit of 100 millirem (1 milliSieverts) for members of the public.

CHEMICALS IN OUR ENVIRONMENT
AND IN OUR FOOD

Exposure to natural and human-made chemicals in the environment accounts for two-thirds of cancer. The amount of chemical carcinogens that people are exposed to varies greatly. Some people are exposed to high concentrations of chemicals in their workplace. Others are exposed to common household carcinogens or natural carcinogens depending on where they live.

The way many substances act as a carcinogen is a matter of chemistry. Many chemicals that are carcinogens are electrophiles (electron loving; containing positively charged parts). Since opposites attract, electrophiles search for nucleophiles (containing negatively charged parts), including the bases of DNA. As a result, chemical carcinogens chemically bind to DNA. The addition of a chemical to DNA forms a **DNA adduct**. DNA adducts mask the base sequence of DNA. When the cell divides, its sequence cannot be read properly and as a result an incorrect base may be incorporated into the newly synthesized DNA strand leading to a mutation. This error is passed down in future cell divisions and may produce 'faulty' cell products that contribute to tumor formation.

There are too many chemical carcinogens to name but they can be grouped into at least 10 classes. Two of these, polycyclic aromatic hydrocarbons and alkylating agents, played an important role in our understanding of chemical carcinogenesis. Polycyclic aromatic hydrocarbons can be found in coal tar and cigarette smoke. In 1775, a British surgeon named Percival Pott reported the first cancer to be associated with a specific occupation: he observed that scrotal cancer was common in chimney sweeps. The application of coal tar to the ears of rabbits and the subsequent development of skin cancer in 1915 provided early experimental evidence that chemicals could induce cancer. The use of sulfur mustard, also known as mustard gas, during World War I and by Iraqi forces during the Iran–Iraq War of the 1980s, provided insight into alkylating agents as carcinogens. Data from soldiers or civilians exposed to mustard gas demonstrates that this alkylating agent can cause lung cancer (Ghanei and Harandi, 2010). Alkylating agents work by sticking (binding) to DNA directly. The DNA sequence is masked and can lead to misreading of the code such that an 'incorrect' base is incorporated into newly synthesized DNA. Such mutations may lead to cancer.

The kitchen is a place where carcinogens can be added to our food. Cooking meats at high temperatures produces carcinogens called heterocyclic amines. In addition, smoked and barbecued meats often contain carcinogens such as polycyclic aromatic hydrocarbons. We can reduce exposure to some carcinogens by thinking about how we prepare our food. Consider oven roasting instead of frying. Or, if frying meat, try to marinate and coat meat with breadcrumbs beforehand. Simple changes may make a significant difference over a lifetime. In addition, common commercial household cleaners may contain carcinogens and this new knowledge underlies the movement towards using less harsh cleaners such as white vinegar, baking soda, and toothpaste. Indeed, both baking soda and toothpaste are good abrasive cleaners.

Aflatoxin is a potent carcinogen that is produced by fungi growing on peanuts and grains during storage. Contaminated sources for food products such as peanut butter could produce carcinogenic foods. The good news is that many countries now screen these foods before processing and consumption of aflatoxin is no longer a danger in these countries.

HAVING A COUPLE OF DRINKS? MAKE THEM NON-ALCOHOLIC

Alcohol was added to the list of carcinogens by the IARC in 2007. Consumption of alcohol is a causal factor in tumors of the upper digestive tract including the mouth, pharynx, larynx, esophagus, and also liver, colorectal, and breast cancers. Chronic drinking of alcohol accounts for about 3.6% (approximately 389,000 cases) of cancer worldwide. The analysis of evidence for the role of alcohol and cancer reported by the World Cancer Research Fund and the American Institute for Cancer Research justifies a recommendation not to drink alcohol. But, these organizations acknowledge that other evidence shows that modest amounts of alcoholic drinks are likely to reduce the risk of coronary heart disease. While acknowledging this, the British Heart Foundation suggests that there are safer ways to protect your heart, like taking more exercise, eating a healthy diet, and stopping smoking. The World Cancer Research Fund recommends that if alcoholic drinks are consumed they should be limited to two drinks a day for men and one a day for women.

How do we know that alcohol causes cancer? The evidence comes from animal studies and also from many epidemiological studies. Rats and mice who receive alcohol in their drinking water developed more tumors than control animals. One French epidemiological study demonstrated that people who drink more than 80 g (about 0.7 liters or a bottle of wine per day) had an 18-fold higher risk of developing cancer of the esophagus. Together, smoking and drinking increase the risk synergistically (more than the sum of the risk of each habit on its own; think of 2+2 = 5). Over a hundred studies have shown that increased intake of alcohol leads to an increased risk of breast cancer. Data suggest that just one alcoholic drink per day causes a 7% increase in the risk of breast cancer.

There are several possible ways that alcohol causes cancer. One mechanism is identical to that of chemical carcinogens and is revealed by looking at the metabolism of alcohol. Alcohol is broken down by an enzyme called alcohol dehydrogenase to form acetaldehyde. Acetaldehyde is a potent carcinogen; it can stick to and bind DNA and cause mutations. Higher levels of acetaldehyde-DNA adducts have been identified in blood cells of drinkers of alcohol compared to controls. Bacteria in saliva receive alcohol from the blood and contribute to acetaldehyde production. This localized elevated production can cause concentrations in saliva to be 10–100 times that of blood and may partially explain why alcohol affects the mouth and surrounding tissues. The role of bacteria is easily illustrated by measuring acetaldehyde concentrations in saliva after an antiseptic mouthwash: a decrease concentration of 30–50% is observed. Other mechanisms of alcohol carcinogenesis include increasing estrogen concentrations (a known risk factor for breast cancer; see below); liver cirrhosis (a risk factor for liver cancer), and oxidative stress.

Not surprisingly, there is an interplay of genes with alcohol-based cancer risks. Since genes code for enzymes involved in alcohol metabolism, individual variations exist. An inherited deficiency in an enzyme that breaks down acetaldehyde, called acetaldehyde dehydrogenase, is common in Asians (40–50%). Patients suffer from facial flushing and nausea after drinking only a small amount of alcohol. Intake of alcohol causes an increased build-up of acetaldehyde so that those with the deficiency have a higher risk of esophageal cancer than those who do not have a deficiency. Genetic variants of other enzymes involved in alcohol metabolism can also affect cancer risk.

The good news is that we can choose to reduce our alcohol consumption, and by doing so reduce cancer risk. Regular and excessive alcohol drinking, like smoking, is out of date. The European Code Against Cancer recommends a maximum daily alcohol intake of 20–30 g (approximately 250 ml or a quarter bottle of wine) for men and half this amount for women. The US Department of Agriculture, and Health and Human Services advise similar alcohol intake, with a maximum of 28 g in men and half this for woman. Since the cancer-causing ingredient in alcoholic drinks is alcohol (ethanol), the recommendations cover all types: beers, wines, and spirits.

ESTROGEN

Steroidal estrogens are listed as a carcinogen by both IARC and the US National Toxicology Program *Report on Carcinogens*. Estrogen is a natural steroid hormone but is also used in oral contraceptives and hormone-replacement therapy. Evidence strongly suggests that increased exposure to estrogen is carcinogenic. It has been observed for hundreds of years that nuns have a higher rate of breast cancer. Epidemiological studies, including the study of over 31,000 catholic nuns published in 1969 by Joseph Fraumeni Jr. and colleagues, confirmed higher rates of breast cancer mortality in nuns. The researchers concluded that the excess of breast cancer mortality was probably mediated by hormones, reflecting the lack of hormone changes that accompany pregnancy. Estrogen levels are lower during pregnancy. Since nuns, in general, do not have children, they have an increased exposure to estrogens and an increased risk of breast cancer.

It may be of interest for women in Western societies who delay having children to later ages to note that late age at first full-term pregnancy is a well-established risk factor for breast cancer. Pregnancy at an early age is protective against breast cancer and its effect is permanent. Hormones associated with pregnancy such as progesterone are involved in the specialization and maturation of tissue in the breast and this maturation process may be one of the protective events of pregnancy.

Hormones are powerful molecules because they activate partner molecules called hormone receptors that can turn on sets of genes. Turning on sets of genes can have a big impact on cell behavior. Estrogen and the estrogen receptor can stimulate the growth of breast cells. This is noticeable during the female monthly reproductive cycle and during pregnancy when breasts increase in size; breasts can nearly double in size during pregnancy. So it is suggested that too much estrogen may be able to cause abnormal growth and increased chance of mutations. Another possible way that estrogens may cause breast cancer is linked to its metabolites. Like alcohol, a breakdown product of estrogen, estradiol 3,4-quinone, is carcinogenic. It can stick to DNA and form DNA adducts. These adducts cause the bases to detach from the DNA and this leads to mutations that may underlie breast cancer development.

Hormone-replacement therapy (HRT) was widely prescribed to women to alleviate some symptoms of menopause. HRT involves the prescription of estrogen or estrogen plus progestin. A significant clinical trial reported that estrogen-plus-progestin HRT leads to a 24% increased risk of breast cancer compared to patients taking a placebo. Estrogen-only HRT results in an increased risk of stroke and blood clots. The news of these clinical trial findings and supporting studies such as the Million Women Study spread among the public and resulted in a decrease in the use of HRT in Australia, the UK, and the USA. A decrease in the number of new cases of breast cancer followed the change in choice.

INFECTIOUS AGENTS: CAN YOU CATCH CANCER?

Several infectious agents (viruses and bacteria) have been classified as carcinogens. But you cannot 'catch' cancer like you can catch a cold. Cancer development from a virus or bacteria requires long-term, chronic infection and includes a series of events in addition to viral or bacterial infection.

Human papillomavirus (HPV) infection is the causative agent of cervical cancer. It is the most common sexually transmitted viral infection. Although it is the causative agent of cervical cancer, most women who are infected by the virus do not develop cervical cancer because the infection is usually short term and is cleared by the immune system. Only long-term infection leads to cervical cancer. Two viral protein products, E6 and E7, are the major players in the process of cancer development. These proteins bind to and block the action of cell proteins whose role is to suppress tumors by regulating cell growth and DNA repair. One of these tumor suppressor proteins is P53. So cells containing E6 and E7 display unregulated growth and accumulate mutations. More recently, evidence has suggested that HPV infection due to oral sex is a causative factor in some head and neck cancers.

Other viruses that are causative agents of cancer include human T-cell leukemia virus type-1 (common in the Caribbean and Japan) which causes adult T-cell leukemia, hepatitis B virus which causes liver cancer, and Kaposi's sarcoma-associated herpes virus which causes Kaposi's sarcoma.

Specific strains of a bacterium, called *Helicobacter pylori*, cause chronic infection of the gut and is a causative agent of gastric cancer. The manner by which this bacterium causes cancer parallels the mechanisms of HPV. That is, bacterial proteins interact with cell proteins and can stimulate growth. Also, *H. pylori* triggers inflammation that creates an environment high in reactive oxygen species, leading to increased rates of mutation.

The good news about our knowledge of viral and bacterial carcinogens is that we can deploy commonly used medical interventions such as vaccines and antibiotics to prevent or treat them.

DEFENSE SYSTEMS

We have several remarkable defense systems against damage caused by carcinogens, and ultimately tumors. One defense system is detoxifying enzymes in the liver that modify carcinogens for rapid removal. The family of enzymes called the cytochrome P450 enzymes chemically alter many fat-soluble carcinogens to become water-soluble so that they can be easily excreted. Interestingly, the activity of some members of this enzyme family can vary up to 50-fold among individuals and therefore can account for some people being more susceptible to the effects of carcinogens compared to other individuals.

Another important defense against carcinogens is DNA repair. Cells can sense and recognize several different types of DNA damage such as UV-induced pyrimidine dimers, DNA adducts, and DNA strand breaks. Subsequently, protein factors are recruited to the site of damage and through a series of steps can physically cut out (remove) the damaged portion of DNA and fill in the missing piece such that the molecule is returned to its original sequence. A variety of DNA-repair enzymes are involved in this process. The DNA sequence that is removed is precisely replaced using the specific base-pairing rule (A–T; C–G) and the opposite strand as a template, as in DNA replication (Figure 4). DNA repair is co-ordinated with a pause in cell division so that DNA damage does not lead to errors during DNA replication and this avoids mutation.

Evidence that DNA-repair systems play a crucial role in our defense against carcinogens is provided by the consequences of genetic defects in these systems. For example, people who have the inherited disorder called xeroderma pigmentosum have a deficiency in an enzyme involved in the repair of UV-induced damage. These patients are hypersensitive to the sun and have a 1000-fold-increased risk of skin cancer. Another inherited disorder called Lynch syndrome (also known as hereditary nonpolyposis colorectal cancer, or HNPCC) involves a defect in DNA-repair proteins and is one of the most common cancer syndromes in humans. Patients have about a 70% lifetime risk of colon cancer.

If you thought that DNA repair is a clever defense system, the one described next is even more extreme. In brief, if cells receive so much damage that the cell is unable to repair the DNA, a genetic program is triggered that results in cell suicide. That is, rather than risking that a cell containing a large amount of DNA damage may become cancerous, the cell is instead eliminated for the good of the whole individual. This process was described as a reaction to sunburn. The process of cell suicide is precise and tidy. It should not be confused with other forms of cell death that occur in response to cell injury that causes explosion of cell contents into the surrounding area leading to inflammation.

Tumor suppressor proteins play a major role in the defense systems against tumors. P53 is a 'star player' in tumor suppression and plays a role in the production of detoxifying enzymes, DNA repair, pausing cell division, and cell suicide (Figure 8). But *how* does P53 orchestrate these cell actions? The power of P53 is mainly due to its role as a **transcription factor**. That is, it is able to bind to the controlling regions of sets of genes and turn them either on or off. In the absence of cell stress the P53 turns on genes whose products are involved in antioxidant activities. These genes code for detoxifying enzymes that are involved in the metabolism of reactive oxygen species. P53 turns on genes that produce DNA-repair enzymes in response to DNA damage, including enzymes involved in repairing UV damage. At the same time P53 turns on genes that produce proteins that bind and block proteins needed for cell division. This allows time to repair the DNA before the DNA is replicated. Extensive DNA damage will cause P53 to turn on a different set of genes whose products are involved in cell suicide. One such gene product causes the release of specific enzymes stored in the mitochondria of cells that chew up proteins. These enzymes, called caspases, digest components of the cell and allow for its disassembly and eventual removal by

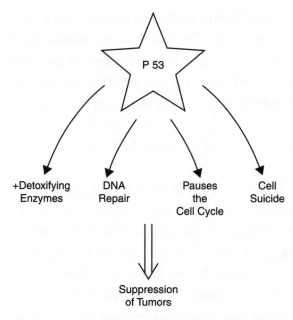

FIG 8 How does the P53 tumor suppressor block the formation of tumors?

immune cells called macrophages. For example, caspases digest proteins that support the nuclear membrane and the skeleton proteins of the cell. They also trigger the digestion of DNA into small fragments.

A faulty P53 system, caused by mutation, gives opportunity for tumors to form and so it may not be surprising to hear that the P53 system is altered in most cancers. Inheritance of a *p53* gene mutation causes Li–Fraumeni syndrome, a condition characterized by a 25-fold increased risk of developing a wide range of cancers before 50 years of age.

In addition to DNA damage, abnormal growth signals and low oxygen levels (discussed in chapters ahead) are stress conditions that support tumors and trigger P53 into action. There are many other tumor suppressor genes, such as the retinoblastoma (Rb) gene and the BRCA1 gene, involved in the regulation of cell division and DNA repair respectively, that are part of our army of tumor suppressors. Isn't it fascinating how our body strives to protect us?

THE GOOD NEWS

The good news is that public awareness about carcinogens is spreading and, increasingly, people are choosing to change their lifestyle to avoid or decrease exposure to them. Lifestyle is a matter of choice. The dangers of excessive sunbathing and the use of sunscreen lotions is one example of how knowledge has led to changes in lifestyle habits. The decrease in the use of HRT after the findings of clinical trials and the subsequent decrease in breast cancer is another piece of good news. Spreading the word that alcohol is a carcinogen is taking root and promises to make a difference as people choose to limit their intake and choose different options. Sharing non-alcoholic drinks can be an alternative social activity and places like coffee shops have provided a comfortable environment for non-alcoholic socializing. Keeping a watch on how to protect the integrity of your genes is an important way to reduce cancer risk.

4

ALL WE HAD TO DO
WAS QUIT

In the future, the greatest reductions in cancer-associated mortality
will come from preventing the disease rather than treating it once
it has been detected. Changes in lifestyle will prove vastly more
important than novel treatments of the disease.

Robert Weinberg, Professor for Cancer Research, Whitehead Institute,
Massachusetts Institute of Technology

Christopher Columbus and his crew learned about tobacco
leaves that were presented to them by natives of the New World
in October 1492 and are credited as the first people to bring tobacco
to Europe soon after. Up until and during the 19th century, smokers
generally used pipes or cigars. And then came the cigarette.

The fashion of smoking cigarettes exploded in the USA and
Europe during and after World Wars I and II, when cigarettes were
manufactured for large-scale consumption. The trend began first
among men and then among women. In the second half of the 20th
century smoking spread throughout the world. Smoking became
cool, glamorous, calming for the nerves, and a contagious social

activity. We all know the images: the Marlboro Man in his blue jeans against the backdrop of the Wild West, Greta Garbo with her 12-inch cigarette holder, and, for the average mortal, morning coffee, the newspaper, and a cigarette. Nicotine contained within the tobacco made smoking addictive.

Now we know better. Smoking is a causative factor of lung cancer. Lung cancer is the leading cause of cancer-related death in the world (over 1 million deaths per year). Cigarette smoking causes about 90% of lung cancer cases in men in the USA. But it took some time to prove, hear, and understand the fact that smoking causes cancer. It was time that showed us that Wayne McLaren, one of the Marlboro Men, would die of lung cancer at age 51. Members of royalty affected included King George VI of England, who died of lung cancer at the age of 56, and 'US Royal' Jackie Kennedy Onassis, a closet chain smoker, at 64.

The scientific proof began to accumulate in the mid-20th century. Several studies published in 1950 examined the smoking history of patients with lung cancer and *suggested* that tobacco smoking was linked to lung cancer. These studies compared the smoking habits of patients with lung cancer to those without. This type of study is called a retrospective case-control study because it looks back over time. Stronger evidence would be provided by large prospective studies following smokers and non-smokers forward over time into the future. One landmark prospective study, carried out by Richard Doll and Austin Bradford Hill, examined the mortality of British doctors in relation to smoking and confirmed a link between smoking and lung cancer in the UK (Doll and Hill, 1954). Another landmark prospective study, carried out by Harold Dorn, examined US veterans over a two-and-a-half year period and also concluded that there was a causal link between smoking and lung cancer. In the early 1960s the US Surgeon General and the UK Royal College of Physicians affirmed that smoking leads to lung cancer and soon afterwards legislation was passed to ensure warning labels were printed on all cigarette packs. Cigarette advertisements started to disappear. Similar steps were taken in the UK. These actions began to convey the seriousness of smoking in the UK and USA. Between 1950 and 1990 the prevalence of smoking in UK men had been halved and is still decreasing (Figure 9): very good

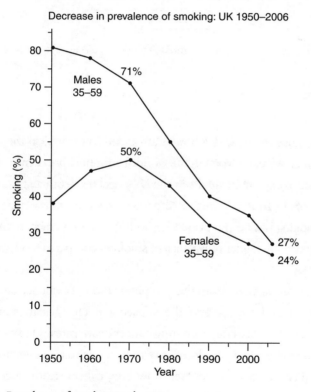

Decrease in prevalence of smoking: UK 1950–2006

FIG 9 Prevalence of smoking in the UK, 1950–2006.

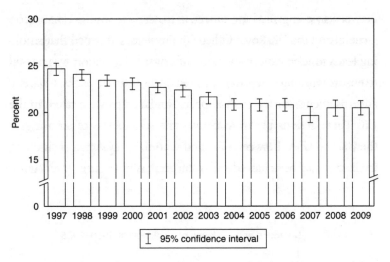

FIG 10 Prevalence of current smoking among adults aged 18 years and over in the USA, 1997–2009.

news, since the male death rates attributed to tobacco in the UK in the 1960s were the worst in the world. The annual prevalence of current smoking among adults in the USA declined from 24.7% in 1997 to 20.6% in 2009 (Figure 10). Although a decrease in the prevalence of smoking has been reported for both men and women, men have a significantly higher prevalence of smoking compared to women in the USA.

So, after 60 years from the first publication of evidence between smoking and cancer and the subsequent changes in smoking habits, can we see effects on lung cancer death rates? Oh yes, there is good news. And you don't have to be a scientist to interpret the data (Plate 2). See for yourself how lung cancer death rates have fallen in the USA over recent years.

Some attempts at decreasing the harmful effects of cigarette smoking were less successful. Changes in cigarette design were aimed at trying to reduce the amount of tar delivered and filter-tip cigarettes were created. Ninety-seven percent of the cigarettes sold in the US today are filtered. Filters are usually made of cellulose, although some early filters used asbestos, another lung carcinogen! Some filters in 'light' cigarettes are perforated on the sides with tiny holes. The holes allow air through the filter to dilute the smoke inhaled. The theory is that the smoker will be exposed to less tar. A report published by the National Cancer Institute has concluded that evidence does not indicate an important health benefit from changes in cigarette design over the last 50 years. The results of the National Cancer Institute report may be explained by how these cigarettes are smoked. People who smoke filtered low-tar cigarettes seem to take more puffs and inhale more deeply to compensate for the reduced delivered tar. Some smokers even block the ventilation holes with their fingers or lips while inhaling. People are misled into thinking that the low-tar cigarettes are less dangerous and are discouraged from smoking cessation. The verdict from many studies is that filter ventilation is a dangerous and defective technology that should be abandoned. There is no such thing as a safe cigarette. The decrease in lung cancer deaths seen in Plate 2 is due to the decrease in smoking prevalence and is not due to changes in cigarette design.

Towards the end of the 20th century another critical step was taken to help people 'kick the habit'. In 1990, a city in California, called San Luis Obispo, set an example for the world and became the first place in the world to ban smoking in public buildings. I am currently living in London, UK, almost half way around the world from this city, and have watched the wave of smoking bans travel across America, and just recently arrive in Northern Europe. We await its spread to China where people currently behave as if they have not heard the news that smoking causes cancer. Unfortunately, lung cancer rates are rising in China. The BBC news reported that a Chinese county has ordered civil servants and teachers to smoke locally made cigarettes in the hopes of boosting the local economy via cigarette tax. A large study of over 169,000 Chinese adults, published by Gu et al., in the *New England Journal of Medicine* in 2009, concluded that smoking is a major risk factor for mortality in China and suggests that national smoking prevention and cessation campaigns are needed. In contrast, smoking is not a social activity in Kenya and lung cancer is not within the top five types of cancer incidence.

It is the banning of smoking in public places, with its consequence that people quit smoking, that may become one of the most influential acts against cancer. And it's not just former smokers who may benefit. In 1986, the US Surgeon General concluded that environmental tobacco smoke causes lung cancer in adults. Later on the US Environmental Protection Agency estimated that environmental tobacco smoke causes 3000 lung cancer deaths a year among American non-smokers. Smoking bans decrease the exposure of second-hand smoke to non-smokers as well as causing changes in the behavior of smokers. The International Agency for Research on Cancer (IARC) published its study (IARC, 2009) on the effectiveness of smoke-free policies. It concluded that:

1. There is sufficient evidence that smoke-free workplaces decrease cigarette consumption in continuing smokers.

2. There is sufficient evidence that implementation of smoke-free policies substantially decreases second-hand smoke exposure.

3. There is strong evidence that smoke-free policies decrease tobacco use in youths.
   (From IARC, 2009)

There are numbers to back claims of effectiveness. For example, in the UK the Smoking Toolkit study estimated that 400,000 people quit smoking in the first year after the ban began in summer 2007. Banning smoking in public places has made an impact on the personal lifestyles of many. Non-smokers are enjoying places such as pubs, bars, and restaurants that were previously tainted by smoke. It will take a few decades to see the consequences of the smoking bans on lung cancer because it takes several decades for lung cancers to develop. Smoking bans are likely to be the reason behind further good news with regards to decreasing lung cancer deaths in the future.

The concept that there is no such thing as a safe cigarette must be kept at the center of objectives as the US Food and Drug Administration (FDA) exerts its newly gained power to regulate cigarettes and other tobacco products. Signed into law by President Obama, the Family Smoking Prevention and Tobacco Control Act of 2009 has given this regulatory authority to the FDA to protect the health of the public. Under the leadership of Commissioner Margaret Hamburg, the FDA has banned flavored cigarettes, so as not to entice the young smoker. It is now illegal in the USA to buy fruit-, candy-, clove-, and chocolate-flavored cigarettes. A federal minimum age of 18 years for buying cigarettes has been set. There is a ban on the distribution of free samples of cigarettes and brand-name sponsorship for sporting events and concerts by tobacco companies is prohibited. The power of the FDA to analyze ingredients in cigarettes may lead to additional bans on various types of cigarettes. Stronger health warnings on cigarette labels and in marketing campaigns are actions that the FDA may impose in the near future that could have a positive impact. The regulation of tobacco by the FDA presents an historic opportunity to make a huge impact on public health by applying their regulatory expertise and experience from the food and drug fields.

SO HOW DOES SMOKING CAUSE CANCER?

A friend smoked before getting breast cancer. She has been treated and has remained disease-free for five years. Yet she still smokes. When asked whether she believed smoking causes cancer, she replied 'no'. This is a person who has had a mastectomy. She is fully aware of cancer as a disease but she does not understand her role in preventing a second type of cancer, lung cancer. Some people still do not believe that cigarette smoking causes lung cancer. This is regrettable, because the mechanism is clear and the scientific evidence is rock solid.

Cigarette smoke contains not one, but *eighty one* different carcinogens, as classified by the International Agency on Cancer. Nicotine, although addictive, is not a carcinogen. Let's just examine one of the 81 carcinogens. The most well-known chemical carcinogen in cigarette smoke is benzo[a]pyrene. It is also one of the most potent mutagens identified. Inhalation of cigarette smoke creates a direct route for the carcinogen to lung cells. The chemical structure of benzo[a]pyrene allows it to enter cells easily. It travels to the nucleus of the cells and sticks to DNA. Nitrosamines and nitrosamides are additional types of carcinogens found in tobacco smoke. They mainly stick to Gs in DNA. This chemical addition to our DNA (DNA adducts) acts to mask the genetic code. As a result, the genetic instructions are not copied correctly when a cell reproduces and a permanent error is made in the DNA. This error is then passed down to all subsequent daughter cells and results in the making of 'faulty' cell products. And faulty cell products that control cell growth can lead to abnormal cell growth in a group of cells, causing the creation of a tumor (Figure 11). The physical presence of a tumor in a lung, among other things, makes it difficult to breathe.

It is estimated that 40% of **all** cancer mortality is attributed to exposure to tobacco smoke (this represents 1.18 million deaths

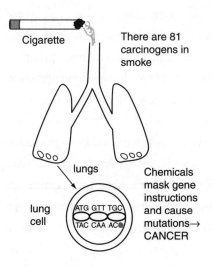

Cigarette

There are 81 carcinogens in smoke

lungs

lung cell

ATG GTT TGC
TAC CAA AC

Chemicals mask gene instructions and cause mutations→ CANCER

FIG 11 How does smoking cause cancer? Particles in smoke enter the cells of your lungs and stick to and mask the instructions of your genes. This leads to permanent damage of your genes (mutations) that get passed down to all daughter cells. Mutations in genes that are involved in growth can lead to a lung tumor.

annually). It is obvious why smoking causes lung cancer: cigarette smoke is inhaled directly into the lungs. It may be not as obvious that cigarette smoking is also associated with mouth cancer and cancer of the larynx, pharynx, esophagus, stomach, liver, pancreas, kidney, bladder, and ureter. These are tissues that become exposed as the carcinogens enter and leave the body.

A landmark study by Gerd Pfeifer and his colleagues, carried out in the Beckman Research Institute of the City of Hope, California, in 1996, provided molecular evidence for the role of benzo[a]pyrene in lung cancer. The study focused on the *p53* gene, which is mutated in 60% of lung cancers. The mutations observed in tumors are located in particular places within the gene, called hotspots. Although the *p53* gene may be mutated in other cancers, one mutational hotspot is specific for lung cancer. Pfeifer's team investigated whether the same mutations observed in lung cancer patients could be reproduced in the laboratory by exposing lung cells to benzo[a]pyrene. They exposed human lung cells to benzo[a]pyrene and then mapped the exact positions of the 'masks' or DNA adducts on the *p53* gene. Since hundreds of DNA base pairs were analyzed, all of which are possible targets for mutation, matching profiles would be strong evidence that they were caused by the same agent. (Just imagine asking two people to randomly pick out three letters from the alphabet; it would be very unlikely that two people would choose the same letters; and this is only from a set of 26 letters.) They found that the location of DNA adducts precisely matched the location of mutations found in lung tumors from smokers. Pfeifer's results provide strong evidence that benzo[a]pyrene in cigarette smoke causes lung cancer.

It is important to explain why some people live long lives smoking many cigarettes per day. Indeed, these exceptions make great headlines: World Oldest Man Celebrates 115th Birthday; quit 76-year smoking habit at 90 (August 22, 2006, Associated Press). Such statements make great headlines because they are really anomalies. Large studies have shown that non-smokers live longer. Take the study of 15,000 men and women carried out over 28 years conducted by Laurence Gruer and colleagues at the University of Glasgow, and published in 2009. From their results they concluded that smokers of all social classes ran a much higher risk of dying early than non-smokers. So the one habit of not smoking, rather than money or social class, has a major influence if you want to live a long life. Sir Richard Doll and his colleagues have calculated that, on average, cigarette smokers die about 10 years younger than non-smokers. These data, published in 2004, come from a 50-year-long (1951–2001) prospective follow-up study of mortality in relation to smoking among British doctors born between 1900 and 1930. On average, these men started smoking at 18 years of age and smoked about 20 cigarettes per day. As one may appreciate, this type of data is not easy to obtain due to the long time period needed to evaluate life expectancy but it is extremely valuable and relevant for predicting future mortality trends based on current smoking patterns.

An explanation for the exceptions to the rule lies within a person's genes. The body's defense system for dealing with carcinogens involves a number of enzymes that modify the carcinogens for excretion. Paradoxically, some of the reactions create more potent intermediates before reaching a product ready for removal. Small variations in enzyme activities, dictated by our genes, can help explain why some smokers may escape the extent of cellular damage required for triggering lung cancer. Another explanation is pure chance. Remember that mutations in genes that control cell number give rise to cancer but mutations in many other genes may not contribute to cancer formation. But what a risky game to play!

Genes may help to explain why some people become addicted to nicotine whereas others do not. Genome-wide studies have discovered genetic variations on chromosome 15 associated with lung cancer. Some scientists believe that a gene in the specified region produces protein receptors that have affinity for nicotine. So genetic variation may explain why some people get addicted to cigarettes while others do not; it may influence how many and how often people smoke. Note that these receptors normally bind to chemical messengers of neurons, called neurotransmitters. Nicotine has a similar shape to a specific neurotransmitter that plays a role in reward pathways related to life-sustaining activities and results in happy, pleasant feelings. Ironically, nicotine produces pleasurable sensations to smoking, a life-shortening activity. In the future, knowledge of an individual's genome, including genes that determine nicotine dependence, may be useful in helping to kick the habit.

Is smoking marijuana (cannabis) less harmful than smoking cigarettes? The current evidence is not clear for several reasons, including the fact that it is difficult to get large data sets on the use of an illegal substance. It is also difficult to separate the effects of marijuana from the effects of tobacco since many people smoke both, and tobacco may be mixed with marijuana (a custom in the UK). The facts remain that marijuana contains at least 50 of the

81 carcinogens present in cigarettes, filters do not tend to be used during the smoking of marijuana, and most smokers of marijuana inhale more deeply. Although there is some evidence that one constituent (delta-9-tetrahydrocannabinol) may have anti-tumor effects, the writing is on the wall. Data from a recent case-control study carried out on a distinct population (New Zealand) where marijuana is rarely mixed with tobacco suggest that long-term cannabis smoking increases the risk of lung cancer in young adults (Aldington et al., 2008). These researchers estimate that for each joint-year of cannabis use the risk of lung cancer increases by 8%. The potential cancer-causing effects must be noted during debates about the legalization of marijuana use. Support for the proposal to legalize marijuana is strong in California. Wouldn't it be ironic if California, the first state to ban cigarette smoking, turns out to be the first state to legalize marijuana? Two steps forward and one step back?

Non-smokers can get lung cancer. Some scientists believe that particular genetic variations are associated with inherited susceptibility to lung cancer, similar to the BRCA1 and BRCA2 genes for breast cancer. Studies of family histories and lung cancer incidence support the role for genetic factors in lung cancer. An individual who has a first-degree relative diagnosed with lung cancer before the age of 60 has a five-fold increased risk of getting lung cancer before 60 years. Early-onset cases of lung cancer suggest that genetic factors may play a role in causation. There are molecular differences between lung tumors from non-smokers and smokers that define distinct tumor etiology and biology. Understanding these differences will inform better treatment choices in the future.

OTHER LUNG CARCINOGENS

Asbestos and radon gas are two other causative agents for lung cancer. Asbestos is a group of naturally occurring fibrous minerals. Asbestos was used as insulation in the building industry before it was prohibited due to its classification as a carcinogen. It is a causative factor for lung cancer and mesothelioma. Mesothelioma is cancer of the mesothelium, a protective membrane that covers most of the internal organs of the body. Interestingly, those with extensive exposure to asbestos and cigarette smoke have an enhanced increased risk of cancer, larger than the sum of each risk alone.

Erionite, like asbestos, is also a naturally occurring fibrous mineral that is carcinogenic. It can be found in certain volcanic rocks. Small isolated geographical locations in Turkey have epidemics of malignant mesothelioma, where 50% of all deaths are due to this cancer. Scientists were puzzled why some villages in erionite-rich regions had epidemics of mesothelioma and others did not. Perhaps different types of erionite were present, where one type caused mesothelioma and one type did not. Physical and chemical tests proved this was not the case. Family pedigrees revealed that there is a genetic factor that predisposes individuals to mineral-fiber carcinogenesis. That is, a gene is responsible for susceptibility to an environmental cancer-causing factor. Different fates of individuals having similar exposures to carcinogens become understandable when we factor in genetics.

Radon is an invisible lung carcinogen. Some houses that people live in are like radioactive gas chambers because they trap radon-222, a gas produced from uranium-238 found within the earth's crust beneath the floor. Radon is commonly released from foundations of granite rock across the globe but it is only harmful in enclosed spaces. The radon decays and results in the emission of radiation. Recently, adverts sponsored by the Environmental Protection Agency (http://epa.gov/radon) have been posted in public places to raise the awareness of the importance of radon-resistant homes to help protect against lung cancer. In the USA, 7% of houses have dangerously elevated levels of radon. Data from one study estimated that radon in homes accounts for 2% of all deaths from cancer in Europe (Darby et al., 2005). The good news is that existing buildings can be modified fairly cheaply to reduce radon concentrations and new buildings can be specifically constructed to prevent this occurrence by installing a radon-proof barrier at ground level. Reference to maps that indicate the location of areas in the UK and the USA with the potential for elevated indoor radon levels are listed in the bibliography.

THE GOOD NEWS

Lung cancer is a deadly cancer. Early detection of lung cancer is rare. Treatment is difficult and **prognosis** is poor. Most (though not all) lung cancers have an environmental cause and we know the major culprit. The good news is that most lung cancer can be avoided by not smoking. Education is key, to discourage smoking in those who have not yet started. More good news is that stopping smoking works. If you stop smoking at 40 years of age, you generally only lose one year of life expectancy instead of 10 years (mentioned above). If you stop earlier than 40 years of age, life expectancy is even better. Even stopping smoking at 60 years of age rather than continuing to smoke gains three years of life expectancy, on average. The message is: stop smoking. Kicking the habit is not easy because it is a true addiction caused by nicotine. More good news is that the list of FDA-approved pharmacological agents that help those who are attempting to stop smoking is growing. These include nicotine-replacement treatments (such as Champix/Chantix; made by Pfizer) and a particular antidepressant called bupropion SR (Wellbutrin or Zyban; made by GlaxoSmithKline; available on prescription only). The UK is a model of good practice in that it is the only country in the world that has a network of free stop-smoking services, recently supported by specialized training for the National Health Service Stop Smoking practitioners.

5

TOO MUCH
OF A GOOD THING

We don't know everything but we know enough to intervene
therapeutically and learn from experience.

*Paul Workman, Director of Cancer Research UK Centre for Cancer
Therapeutics, Institute of Cancer Research*

Have you ever wondered about the difference between a table or chair and a living thing? One difference between the living and non-living is the ability for living things to reproduce. The building block of life, the cell, reproduces by cell division. Cell division, also called cell growth, relates to an increase in cell number in this context and not cell size. Cell growth allows tissues to form and regenerate themselves. Cell growth enabled us to develop into an individual with trillions of cells from a single cell, the fertilized egg. In an adult, cell growth is also important in the healing of wounds.

One of the defining characteristics of cancer is that it exhibits uncontrolled cell growth. A description of the events required for controlled cell growth in healthy individuals may help us to understand how uncontrolled growth occurs in cancer.

Cell growth is a highly regulated process. It has to be. Although cell growth happens daily, we maintain our size and form. Cell growth must be balanced with cell death and cell specialization in order to keep the net number of cells in our body more or less constant. We can see controlled growth in the skin, a tissue that constantly regenerates and heals itself from frequent abrasions. Most cells in the body are not continually reproducing. Cell growth requires specific protein signals, called growth factors, which are present on the outside of the cell. These growth factors fit into receptors on the cell membrane like a key fitting into a lock. The signal is passed along a chain of carrier molecules inside of the cell into the nucleus. The ultimate target of a growth factor signal is to regulate a specific set of genes, whose products are needed for cell division.

For example, when a cell divides it requires structural proteins that will pull the chromosomes to opposite ends of the cells so that the cells receive equal amounts of DNA. The genes that code for these structural proteins are turned on by transcription factors that are activated by the growth signal. So a growth pathway generally involves four types of proteins: growth factors, receptors, signal carriers, and transcription factors that initiate, carry, and execute the growth signal. It's like relaying a message along a chain of command; from the leading sergeant through to the corporals, and on to the soldiers who will put the order into action.

Let's explore the molecular details of a one of the most studied growth factor signaling pathways: the EGF signaling pathway. It will be an advantage for you, the reader, if you can actively learn the pathway. There are several reasons for this. It will provide you with a framework to understand many other different types of signaling pathways central to cancer. It will illustrate exactly how a mutation can lead to abnormal growth. Most rewardingly, it will allow an understanding of the rationale and mechanisms of new molecular therapies. Take the challenge at the end of the section and see if you are able to draw the entire pathway.

The star of the show is the growth factor, EGF (which stands for epidermal growth factor). Most molecular nicknames are three or four letters long and if their last two letters are GF, it is usually a growth factor. PDGF, VEGF, FGF are other growth factors.

EGF is the 'key' in this pathway and binds to its 'lock', the EGF receptor. Like a lock that spans the thickness of a door, the EGF receptor spans the cell membrane. There is a part on the outside of the cell, a part that is embedded in the membrane, and a part that lies inside of the cell. The receptor changes shape when it binds to EGF. The change in shape causes two receptors to form a pair, or dimer, and as a result each receptor activates the other.

The activation of proteins in a cell can occur by several mechanisms but one common and important way is modification of a protein by adding a chemical group. The addition of a chemical group causes a change in shape of the protein and this switches it 'on' or 'off'. The chemical group is like an accessory, such as an umbrella. The addition of an umbrella changes the overall shape of a man who holds it above his head and allows him to walk in the rain. In the case of the EGF receptor, the accessory is a phosphate group (indicated by a P in Figure 12) that is added by an enzyme called a **kinase**. The addition of a phosphate group is called **phosphorylation**. The EGF receptor itself is a kinase that is able to phosphorylate target proteins inside of the cell.

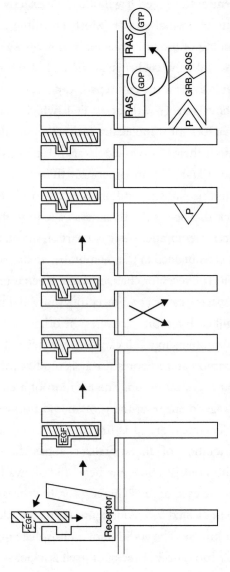

FIG 12 The early steps of the EGF pathway. The EGF growth factor binds to its receptor and causes the receptor to change shape. The change in shape allows two receptors to come together. They phosphorylate each other, shown by a P. The phosphorylated receptor attracts GRB and SOS proteins needed to activate RAS in the membrane. Activation occurs by the replacement of GDP with GTP.

The receiver with its new accessory phosphate 'looks different' and attracts other molecules (e.g. GRB2, SOS) to the cell membrane, like tourists to a tour guide with an umbrella. The recruitment of these molecules in turn activates an important protein embedded in the membrane, named RAS. RAS bound to GDP is inactive whereas RAS bound to GTP is active. Activation of RAS occurs by the exchange of GDP with GTP (Figure 12).

Activated RAS passes the signal away from the membrane to signal carriers in the cytoplasm. The first signal carrier, RAF, also a kinase, adds an accessory phosphate to the next signal carrier, MEK. Phosphorylation causes a change in shape and the activation of MEK. Upon activation, MEK, also a kinase, adds an accessory phosphate to the next signal carrier, MAPK. Phosphorylation of MAPK causes a change in protein shape and activation of MAPK. Like the runners in a relay race where the baton is passed from the first runner to the next, the growth signal is passed through the cell. Activated MAPK, also a kinase, enters the nucleus and ultimately adds an accessory phosphate to a transcription factor. The transcription factor becomes activated and it initiates the expression of a set of genes needed for growth (Figure 13).

The growth signal is transient and is terminated by further modification of the receptor to inhibit its kinase activity. The receptor is also recruited from the cell surface into the cell where it cannot interact with growth signals.

Take a few minutes to look at Figures 12 and 13. Now take the challenge: can you draw the entire EGF signaling pathway? Check your answer. Note the important role of kinases in the growth pathway. They will become important targets for new cancer drugs, discussed below.

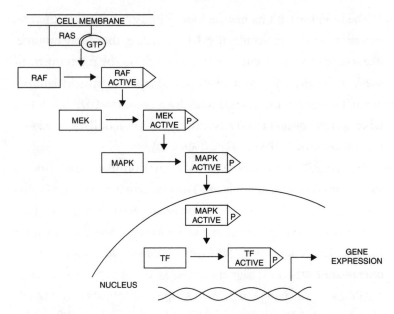

FIG 13 The later steps of the EGF pathway. Activated RAS activates signal carrier RAF, RAF phosphorylates and activates MEK, MEK phosphorylates and activates MAPK, and MAPK enters the nucleus and phosphorylates and activates transcription factors (TF) that turn on specific sets of genes needed for cell growth.

THE DISCOVERY OF ONCOGENES

So why do cancer cells exhibit uncontrolled growth? The answer is simple: mutated genes produce proteins that do not function properly in the growth signaling pathway. How we made this discovery is fascinating and mainly came from work on viruses, simple infectious agents that act as cellular parasites and which are composed of only DNA or **RNA** (that is, ribonucleic acid) and a protein shell.

In 1911, an American scientist named Peyton Rous conducted pioneering work on chicken viruses at the Rockefeller Institute,

New York. He was curious about the cause of sarcomas in chickens. He removed a sarcoma from a chicken and ground up the tissue so that all the cells were destroyed. He then passed the material through a Berkefeld filter that could retain bacteria but not viruses. He then injected the resulting cell filtrate into healthy chickens. Sarcomas appeared in the injected animals. The causative agent from tumors that could transfer cancer to healthy animals was identified as a virus which now bears his name, the Rous sarcoma virus. Years later, scientists discovered that only one viral gene was necessary to cause the cancer. The gene was called *src* and was the first oncogene, a gene involved in the initiation of cancer, to be identified. Interestingly, the gene product was a kinase. Rous was awarded the Nobel Prize in Physiology or Medicine in 1966 for his research.

Sixty years after Rous's experiment, J.M. Bishop and H. Varmus made a surprising discovery which really clinched our current understanding of cancer. They found a gene similar to the viral *src* gene in healthy chicken cells. And even more astonishing to them was that a similar gene was found in organisms throughout the evolutionary tree from flies to humans. The question that demanded an answer was: 'what are they doing in the normal genome?' Their studies led to the conclusion that cancer-causing viruses contain mutated versions of normal cellular genes. The life cycle of some viruses, including the integration of viral DNA into host cellular DNA, allows for the viral genome to recombine, often imprecisely, with host DNA or RNA, leading to the capture of new (altered) genes. This process is known as viral transduction. The importance of Bishop and Varmus' findings is that it provided the molecular link between mutations and cancer, and this is the foundation of our current understanding of cancer biology. The link between cancer and viruses is less important, since 80% of human cancers are not caused by an infectious agent as far as we know. Bishop and Varmus received the Nobel Prize in Physiology or Medicine in 1989 for their work.

We now know that most oncogenes are altered forms of normal cellular genes. Normal genes that *can* be mutated to become oncogenic are called proto-oncogenes. I have often been asked the question, 'cancer is really inside everyone, isn't it?' And although strictly speaking the answer is 'no', I can see where the idea has come from: proto-oncogenes are present in everyone. Carcinogens cause cancer because they cause alterations or mutations of proto-oncogenes that result in oncogenes. These mutations act in a dominant manner (mutation of only one of the two copies of a gene, an **allele,** is needed for the effect) and lead to an increase in activity or gain of function of the oncogene product.

The first role of a proto-oncogene that was discovered was that of a growth factor, called platelet-derived growth factor or PDGF. PDGF is a produced by platelets in response to a wound. Its role is to stimulate cell growth around the wound to facilitate healing and 'fill in' the missing tissue. If the *PDGF* gene is mutated such that it is expressed in abundant quantities or at inappropriate times, one can easily see that this could lead to abnormal cell growth.

THE EGF PATHWAY IN CANCER CELLS

In many cancer cells, mutations affect growth signaling pathways like the EGF pathway. Mutations may affect any of the four types of proteins involved in growth signaling pathways: growth factors, receptors, signal carriers, or transcription factors. In the preceding section we saw that alteration of a growth factor can lead to cancer. A few examples of oncogene activation within the EGF pathway are described below.

The production of oncogenic kinases is common in cancer. Let's look at an example of a mutation that affects the part of the EGF receptor lying on the outside of the cell. The viral oncogenic form of the EGF receptor (also called erbB because it is found in the erythroblastosis virus) has a deletion in the part of the receptor that lies outside of the cell. The mutation causes the receptor to be stuck in the 'always on' mode. That is, it activates the molecular steps described above, even in the absence of the growth factor signal. Think of this as damage to the external face of a lock such that the door always remains open and does not require a key. The effect of this deletion on receptor function has severe consequences: the growth pathway is activated even in the absence of a growth signal. This leads to uncontrolled growth and cancer. Indeed, point mutations that alter the outside part of the EGF receptor have been found in human tumor cells and they have the same consequences as the deletion found in viruses.

Mutations that affect other parts of the EGF receptor, namely the internal part that functions as a kinase, have also been identified in human tumors. Again, affected EGF receptors are stuck in the 'on' position like a jammed switch. The constant phosphorylation of target molecules by the faulty receptor continues to transmit the growth signal and this leads to uncontrolled growth: too much of a good thing.

Mutations in the signal carrier gene, *ras*, are found in 30% of all human tumors. One specific point mutation is common in bladder cancer. The substitution of a T for a G causes an amino acid change from glycine to valine and results in an activated form of RAS protein that is unable to be switched off. As a result, signaling occurs constantly and results in uncontrolled growth.

A transcription factor at the end of the EGF signaling pathway, Fos, is normally precisely regulated. Its gene is turned on in response to growth factors and its mRNA is short-lived so that its protein product functions for a short period. Mutations that transform the *fos* proto-oncogene into an oncogene involve deletion of regulatory sequences that result in extending the life of its mRNA. So more of the protein is made, and since it is a transcription factor its target genes are turned on inappropriately, leading to uncontrolled growth.

We can see from the examples above that mutations in genes that code for many of the proteins involved in growth signaling pathways can contribute to causing cancer.

NEW DRUGS THAT TARGET MOLECULES OF THE EGF GROWTH SIGNALING PATHWAY

This leads us to the application of this scientific information. How can we use our knowledge to create new cancer drugs against the aberrant proteins involved in growth factor signaling? Strategies for designing drugs that target specific steps in the growth signaling pathways become logical when you know 'what is broken'. Any approach that aims to disable the over-active growth signaling pathway has potential. Basically, we need to disable one of the 'relay runners' to break the chain of cell signaling. Let's look at a few examples.

One approach may be to target the EGF receptor since it is mutated in many cancers. A drug could be designed that would bind to the outside part of the receptor. In fact, such a strategy was successful and has resulted in the approval of two drugs called Herceptin (or generic name trastuzumab, in 1998) and Erbitux (or cetuximab, in 2004).

Both Herceptin and Erbitux are scientifically engineered **monoclonal antibodies**. Antibodies are important defense molecules of our immune system that can recognize specific foreign proteins and help the body fight infectious agents such as bacteria and viruses. Herceptin is a drug whose structure is based on our natural antibodies. It is a monoclonal antibody that binds to the outside portion of the EGF receptor and causes it to be brought inside the cell where it is degraded. Let me explain a little more about its name. The EGF receptor is really one of a family of EGF receptors: EGF receptors 1–4. They also have the alternative names of HER1, HER2, HER3, and HER4. Herceptin binds to HER2. The amount of HER2 is high in 30% of breast cancers and so Herceptin is appropriate for the treatment of breast cancer in women whose tumors have abnormally high amounts of HER2 activity. This drug is not effective on cancers that arise from mutations that alter other members of the pathway.

Another strategy is to design a drug that would block the kinase activity present on the part of the EGF receptor that lies inside of the cell. Remember, this activity is important for passing the signal on to molecules inside the cell. This strategy too has been successful and has resulted in the approval of two drugs, called Iressa (the generic name of which is gefitinib) and Tarceva (erlotinib). Iressa has been approved in the European Union since 2009 but has been under limited administration in the USA since 2003. Tarceva was approved in the USA in 2004. The variable response to Iressa is explained in Chapter 13. Drugs that target the EGF receptor are illustrated in Figure 14.

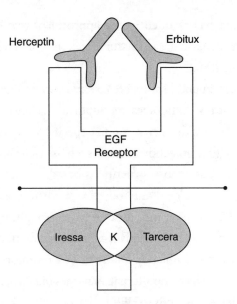

FIG 14 Cancer drugs that target the EGF receptor. Drugs are shaded; 'K' represents the kinase domain of the EGF receptor.

THE GOOD NEWS

The good news is that we are translating our knowledge into new drugs. These drugs target specific molecular defects in cancer cells. This is a positive change from conventional chemotherapies that work by inducing extensive DNA damage to cause cancer cell suicide. Note that many conventional chemotherapies aim to target any rapidly growing cell. They also affect healthy rapidly growing cells, such as hair follicles, cells of the intestines, and blood, causing the all-too-familiar side-effects of losing your hair (alopecia), getting ulcers, and having anemia. The new drugs that target specific molecules promise fewer side-effects, although they are not completely free from them.

6

THE GREAT ESCAPE

We are continually faced with great opportunities which are
brilliantly disguised as unsolvable problems.

Margaret Mead, American anthropologist (1901–1978)

Cancer would not be as lethal if it did not spread throughout
the body. The spread of cancer cells from the original tumor
(**primary tumor**) to distant sites of the body is called **metastasis**,
and it is the major clinical problem that makes cancer difficult to
treat. Ninety percent of cancer-related deaths are due to metastasis. Hippocrates, a Greek physician of the ancient world (c.400 BC),
is credited with the first published description of metastasis. It was
he who named the group of diseases associated with a crab-like
nature and appearance *karkinoma* (carcinoma), the Greek word for
crab. The spread of tumor cells to other parts of the body may
form new metastatic tumors and these tumors may also metastasize and form new tumors. One can easily see why it is crucial
to treat cancer early. The cells in the new metastatic tumors retain
the identity of the cells of the original tumor. For example, when

breast cancer cells metastasize to the brain, the tumor in the brain is made of breast cancer cells and not brain cancer cells. Specific targeting of metastasis is a strategy we can aim for as we delve into a new frontier of the molecular biology of metastasis.

Metastasis can be thought of as a type of great escape. Like all escapes, it is important to understand the terrain through which the escape must occur. Escapes from the prison on the island of Alcatraz must include the ability to separate and move away from other prisoners at the prison, entry into the surrounding sea as a means of transport away from the prison, the ability to survive in the ice-cold turbulent sea, exit from the sea, and the setting up of a new life on the mainland. The prisoner may signal friends for help before he begins his journey. Friends may respond by preparing a shelter for him on the mainland before he arrives. Some escapees may live an isolated life while others may flourish under a new identity. Only a small proportion of attempted escapes are successful because difficulties and failures can be encountered at each step and abort the mission.

Metastasizing tumor cells follow a similar course. It is the acquisition of migratory characteristics by primary tumor cells together with the co-operation of non-tumor cells in the patient that drives the great escape in cancer. Metastasizing cells first detach and move away from the primary tumor. They then enter the bloodstream, a harsh environment for non-blood cells, and move along in one direction according to blood flow. The metastasizing cells leave the bloodstream and set up a new colony at a distant (secondary) site. Recently, scientists have uncovered that non-tumor cells participate in supporting metastasizing cells at a new location after responding to molecular signals from the primary tumor. Some metastasizing cells remain dormant in their new location and others thrive. Only a small proportion are

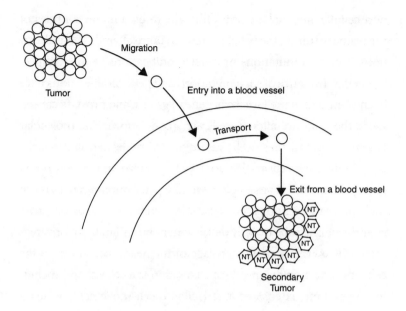

FIG 15 Steps of metastasis. NT, non-tumor cells.

successful, as only 1 in 10,000 metastasizing cells survive the journey. We will take a closer look at the steps of metastasis (Figure 15) above.

EARLY MIGRATION

Most cells of the adult (with the exception of blood and immune cells) remain within a specific organ; skin cells stay in the skin and are not found in the liver and vice versa. Cells have protein links to neighboring cells (e.g. cadherins) and also to non-cellular material in their environment (e.g. integrins). Collagen is an example of a non-cellular material. In order for cells to escape the confines of the primary tumor, the usual protein links are altered. These alterations occur via mutations or other modifications of their respective genes. Evidence of such mutations and gene modifications have been identified in the *E-cadherin* gene in gastric and prostate cancer. Once the links are altered, cells are free to move. The molecular characteristics of these cells resemble the molecular characteristics of migrating cells of the developing embryo. In the developing embryo some cell types originate in one place but migrate to reach their ultimate locations. For example, neural crest cells originate near the neural tube in early development but migrate to form pigment cells of the skin and cartilage of the head. Alterations in the cell's cytoskeleton can produce changes in the cell's shape, including membrane extensions that facilitate cell movement. When a membrane extension protrudes in one direction and the lagging edge of the cell is released the cell moves forward in the direction of the protrusion. Similar to a prisoner who tunnels underground to create an escape route, the cell may create a route to the blood vessels. The cell uses specific proteases (enzymes that cut up proteins) that act as molecular scissors tunneling through its surrounding environment and enable the cell to reach a blood vessel. Scientists have tried to develop drugs that target these specific proteases, but as yet only limited success has been achieved using this strategy.

ENTRY INTO THE BLOOD VESSEL

To gain entry into the bloodstream, the metastasizing cells receive aid from host immune cells called macrophages. This is known because it has been seen, literally. To observe this collaboration between metastasizing cells and host macrophages, John Condeelis and colleagues from the Albert Einstein College of Medicine, New York, captured the 'glow' of jellyfish by isolating the specific jellyfish gene responsible for its fluorescence and used it to label live metastasizing cells. Using multi-photon microscopy, labeled tumor cells can be seen to move towards macrophages near blood vessels. Entry of the tumor cell into the blood vessel by squeezing in between the cells of the blood vessel depends on this association with macrophages. (Movies of this interaction are available within the free reference Wyckoff et al., 2007.)

TRANSPORT

Just like the sea is a treacherous environment for the escaping prisoner, the main route of transport of the metastasizing cell, the bloodstream, is a hostile environment. Sheer forces in an unusual fluid environment often damage the tumor cells. Some metastasizing cells associate with platelets in the blood and form clusters called emboli where they may be more protected compared to single cells. Only a small subset of cells that gain entry into the bloodstream survives. The detection of circulating tumor cells in the bloodstream is being developed for clinical purposes and is discussed in Chapter 10.

EXIT FROM THE BLOOD VESSEL

Exit from a blood vessel involves events similar to entry into a blood vessel. But one additional feature involves the fact that blood vessel cells from different organs express a distinct set of cell surface proteins. These proteins may anchor traveling tumor cells and cause exit at specific sites, supporting the 'seed and soil hypothesis' described in the next section. In other words, complementary molecules, like a magnet and a piece of metal, provide a means for tumors cells to stick to specific locations in blood vessels and this guides their exit.

COLONIZATION: TUMOR GROWTH
AT A DISTANT SITE

The last step of metastasis is the establishment of a progressively growing tumor at a distant site and it requires the formation of new blood vessels (discussed in Chapter 11) to support its growth. Note that even at this late stage in the process some metastasized cells do not thrive but remain dormant for years. Dormancy is a fine balance between cell growth and cell death: overall a state without net growth. Think of this as a sleeping (dormant), distant tumor that has the potential to 'wake up' if the balance is shifted towards growth. Understanding what factors regulate dormancy is a new frontier but progress is being made. If the metastasized tumor is successful at colonization, it too can become a source of metastasizing cells, amplifying the cancer problem.

It is well established that specific cancers metastasize to preferred sites. For example, colon cancer metastasizes to the liver whereas breast cancer metastasizes to the lung and brain. There can be several explanations of why this is true. Pure anatomy explains some of the preferences. Some cancers will metastasize to organs that are closest *en route* via the circulation. This is the case for colon cancers that metastasize to the liver. It is notable that the heart, a constantly pumping organ, is very rarely a site of metastasis.

Metastasis of other cancers does not fit this model but supports the 'seed and soil hypothesis' proposed by Stephen Paget more than a hundred years ago in 1889. This hypothesis is analogous to seeds that only germinate in a particular soil: metastasis depends on the interaction of the cancer cell (seed) with a matched microenvironment (soil). The microenvironment includes the cellular make-up of a tissue, the non-cellular material, and newly arriving cells from other sites. Pairs of molecules, like locks and keys, may provide a way of matching the seed with the soil. Breast cancer cells express a receptor (CXCR4) for a ligand (CXCL12) found in lung cells and supports the seed and soil hypothesis as an explanation for breast cancer metastasis to the lung. Brain metastasis occurs most frequently from breast and lung cancers and is more common than primary brain tumors by 10:1. The blood–brain barrier causes inadequate levels of chemotherapy to reach brain metastasis and so they can be difficult to treat. In some cases of metastasis, both anatomy and molecular determinants play a role. Liver is the first organ downstream from the colon and colon cancer cells preferentially stick to liver cells.

In the analogy used above of the escaping prisoner, the prisoner signals to his friends on the mainland before he begins his journey so that they can prepare a shelter for him that is ready when he arrives. Recently, scientists discovered that cancer cells of the primary tumor release signals that direct host cells to prepare a distant environment for the metastasizing cells. This is called the **premetastatic niche**. As an illustration one may think of the premetastatic niche as a nest built by a bird's mate before she arrives to lay her eggs. How do we know that the premeta-static niche exists? David Lyden and colleagues at Cornell University and Memorial Sloan-Kettering Cancer Center, New York, have used differentially labeled (red and green) cells in mice to show that bone marrow-derived cells (green) arrive and modify a 'soon-to-be' (prospective) metastatic site before tumor cells (red) arrive (Plate 4). In this experiment mice were irradiated to destroy their bone marrow cells. These cells were replaced with green-labeled bone marrow cells via a bone marrow transplant. Such cells are rarely observed in the lungs after this procedure but when tumor cells that usually metastasize to the lungs were injected, the scene changed. Green bone marrow-derived cells appeared in the lungs 12–14 days after tumor cells were injected into the mice. Tumor cells appeared at the metastatic site 4–6 days after the clusters of bone marrow-derived cells appeared. The location of the bone marrow-derived clusters copied the pattern of metastasis of the signaling tumor cells. Similar results were observed when human tumor cells were tested. Tissue-specific patterns of metastasis of some cancers are dictated by signals from the primary tumor that direct the formation of the premetastatic niche at particular locations. Metastasizing cells adhere and grow at these sites.

This is significant because it forces us to look at a bigger picture. The conventional view was that the metastasizing tumor cell was the main and only player and worked in an autonomous manner. Now we have knowledge of molecular signals released from the primary tumor that travel through the body and orchestrate the formation of a 'congenial soil' for metastasis. Experimental evidence suggests that the molecular signals are specific to the type of cancer. Cells grown in culture release signal molecules into the liquid media in which they are grown. If the media from cultured melanoma cells is injected into a mouse, metastasis of a lung carcinoma is redirected to a pattern of metastasis specific for melanoma (spleen and intestine) and follows the establishment of a premetastatic niche at these sites prior to the arrival of tumor cells. These signaling molecules may become targets of drug intervention in the future.

THE NATURE OF THE METASTASIZING CELL

In our analogy of a prison, one can think that the nature of each prisoner is very different. Is it more likely that a convict who has been charged with breaking and entering is more likely to escape than a person who has been convicted for tax evasion? The question could be the basis of a hypothesis. A tumor is a mixture of cells. Scientists have recently detected a small subset of tumor cells called cancer stem cells. Cancer stem cells have some characteristics of stem cells. Cancer stem cells can self-renew and initiate new tumor formation. For example, experimental evidence suggests that about one in a million leukemia cells can give rise to a new leukemia when transplanted into a living host and these cells contain similar molecular profiles to normal blood stem cells. One hypothesis is that cancer stem cells could be the cells that seed metastasis.

As discussed in earlier chapters, the body has mechanisms that block the formation of tumors. Recently, genes whose function involve blocking metastasis, but do not affect the growth of the primary tumor, have been identified. These genes are called **metastasis suppressor genes** and over 20 have been found. In some cases, the loss of activity of a specific metastasis suppressor gene is needed for metastasis to occur. One metastasis suppressor gene called *KISS1*, discovered in Hershey, Pennsylvania, has been shown to be involved in one of the very last steps of metastasis: the transition from a single cell or small group of cells at a distant site to an actively growing metastatic tumor. In other words, KISS1 maintains dormancy of metastasizing cells, preventing the formation of an actively growing metastatic tumor. The mechanism of how KISS1 works is largely unknown. But that has not stopped scientists from trying to exploit this new knowledge towards a new therapeutic. Small clinical trials that administer KISS1 protein have been carried out but results suggest that side-effects may be a concern in males. Further investigations are ongoing to see whether KISS1 will be the 'kiss of death' to metastasis.

THE JOURNEY TAKEN: THE FAST COURSE VERSUS THE SLOW COURSE

The classical view of metastasis presented above implies that metastasis occurs in a stepwise manner. But a dimension of time needs to placed upon this view to account for the different characteristics of metastasis between different cancers. Cancers such as lung and pancreatic cancer show a rapid course of metastasis that affects many organs. In contrast, metastasis from prostate cancer may appear decades after treatment of the primary tumor. The difference between the two may be determined by when the tumor cells acquire the changes needed for successful metastasis. If the changes required occur in cells of the primary tumor, then a rapid course of metastasis may be observed. Colon cancer may take up to 30 years to become malignant, but when the metastatic cascade begins most of the metastatic traits are acquired in the primary tumor and metastasis is rapid. This concept is supported by studies that have shown that gene expression profiles or 'signatures' of the primary tumor for some cancers can be used to predict the risk of metastasis and disease prognosis. For example, a lung metastasis signature has been identified for breast cancer (Minn et al., 2005). In this research, Joan Massagué and colleagues at Memorial Sloan-Kettering Cancer Center in New York have shown that some of the genes in this signature have important functions in both the primary tumor and in the process of metastasis. This evidence helps resolve conceptual conflicts of why genes important in metastasis would be selected for in a primary tumor; some gene products are important for both primary tumor growth *and* metastasis. If genetic changes that only permit invasion and migration occur in the primary tumor and additional time is needed to acquire characteristics for later stages of successful metastasis, such as colonization, then latency will be observed. The site of colonization may also have an influence on the time dimension of metastasis. The genomics of metastasis is a hot research area and promises to yield crucial information for new drugs.

THE STAGE

New evidence suggests that additional variables, such as the genetic background of the individual, may play a role in metastasis. This is not surprising as one recalls that genetic background plays a role in overall cancer susceptibility and notes the involvement of the host in the metastatic process. Host genetic profiles would have an effect in the primary tumor cells (arising from the host), the surrounding primary tumor environment influencing tumor invasion and migration, and premetastatic sites. Small genetic variations may occur in protein cell links or signaling molecules that inhibit or promote metastasis. Experiments in mice have demonstrated that the ability of mammary tumors to metastasize to the lung depends on small genetic differences between mouse strains. This is an area of research that requires further exploration in humans. It may help to identify those more susceptible to metastasis and lead to strategies to prevent it.

THE GOOD NEWS

The good news is that we have begun to dissect the molecular mechanisms of metastasis and now have hope that this knowledge will lead to new drugs that will specifically target metastasis, the crux of the clinical problem in cancer treatment. The identification of molecules involved in different steps of metastasis will allow us to block their function, just as we have done for tumor growth and angiogenesis. As with more recent cancer treatment strategies, antibodies and small molecules can be engineered to target the molecular targets of metastasis and such agents are already being tested in clinical trials. The ability to identify patients at risk of metastasis at diagnosis will help clinicians deliver the best treatment, avoiding harsh treatment regimes in those who don't need it and applying it to those who do.

7

YOU ARE WHAT YOU
EAT (AND DO)

Through our everyday ways of life (eating, drinking,
physical activities) we have an opportunity to reduce
our risk of cancer...the effort is worth it!

*Professor Annie Anderson, University of Dundee Centre
for Research into Cancer Prevention and Screening*

Did you ever consider *why* we eat? It is not just because food
tastes delicious. We eat because food provides five key elements: energy, materials to build other substances that we need
in the body, vitamins and minerals that allow your enzymes to
function, protection against free radicals, and regulators that turn
genes on and off. As a result, eating well is essential for function-
ing at our optimum. We all know this at some level. When we are
not eating properly and not getting enough vitamins, we feel tired
and fatigued. Vitamins are important for the optimum function-
ing of enzymes that are involved in the chemical reactions needed
to get energy from food. The subject of 'why we eat' may not be
something we think about at every meal but it warrants global

awareness because food and nutrition, along with physical activity, play a central role in cancer prevention.

Dietary factors are thought to account for about 30% of cancers in developed countries (see the review by Key et al., 2002). Studies among different populations have shown there are clear differences in the occurrence of different cancers in different geographical locations and a significant proportion of the variation is due to local diet. Observations of migrating populations and changing diet give correlative evidence that supports this statement. For example, first-generation USA-raised Japanese had a higher risk of colon cancer compared to the Japanese population in Japan and the change in diet is a likely explanation (although other reasons may be possible). Since 1960 meat consumption in Japan has increased seven-fold and this has been mirrored by an almost five-fold increase in cases of colorectal cancer.

Diet is very complex to study so we have a long way to go before we fully understand the relationship between diet and cancer. Some diets may increase our risk of getting cancer and others may help prevent cancer. Studies must not only examine *what* is eaten but must also consider the source, storage, and preparation (how the food is cooked) of food, because these parameters make a difference to the effect of the food.

Let's look at a few examples. Plant foods of a particular type may have different compositions depending on the location and soil in which they are grown. Some fish may accumulate carcinogens because of pollution in their local environment. The source of a particular food could influence the overall positive or negative effects on cancer risk.

Food storage changed dramatically during the 20th century. The use of refrigerators greatly reduced our dependence on salting and pickling and in particular the use of cancer-causing nitrites to preserve food. This, in addition to reduced exposure to the bacterium *Helicobacter pylori* due to cleaner living conditions, is linked to a decrease in the incidence of stomach cancer.

Food preparation can also affect the role a food has on the risk of cancer. Cooking meats at high temperature produces carcinogens. Heterocyclic amines (HCAs), some of the most potent mutagens detected, are present in well-done meats. HCAs have been demonstrated to cause cancer in animals. In order to reduce the quantities of carcinogens that we eat, practices such as frying should be replaced by slow cooking methods, such as roasting.

EVIDENCE-BASED RECOMMENDATIONS FOR THE PREVENTION OF CANCER

When it comes to advice about what and what not to eat with respect to cancer and cancer prevention, there is an overwhelming cacophony of voices. The current truths have been separated from the noise in an official report, entitled *Food, Nutrition, Physical Activity, and the Prevention of Cancer: a Global Perspective*, published by the World Cancer Research Fund and the American Institute for Cancer Research (2007). An expert panel of scientists was called upon to review the masses of scientific publications in the field and to critically assess the evidence provided in these publications to make evidence-based recommendations. The term 'evidence-based' should be emphasized as it is the real value of the report. The report is *the* most authoritative source of information in the field and guides governmental policy-making and health professional practices. In fact, a companion report called *Policy and Action for Cancer Prevention*, published by the World Cancer Research Fund and the American Institute for Cancer Research in 2009, recommends action points for several levels of policy-makers and policy 'influencers', such as the media.

The *Food, Nutrition, Physical Activity, and the Prevention of Cancer* report makes 10 general recommendations for the prevention of cancer, which are listed below.

1. Be as lean as possible without becoming underweight.

2. Be physically active for at least 30 minutes every day.

3. Avoid sugary drinks. Limit consumption of energy-dense foods (particularly processed foods high in added sugar, or low in fiber, or high in fat).

4. Eat more of a variety of vegetables, fruits, wholegrains, and pulses such as beans.

5. Limit consumption of red meats (such as beef, pork, and lamb) and avoid processed meats.

6. If consumed at all, limit alcoholic drinks to two for men and one for women a day.

7. Limit consumption of salty foods and foods processed with salt (sodium).

8. Don't use supplements to protect against cancer.

9. It is best for mothers to breastfeed exclusively for up to six months and then add other liquids and foods.

10. After treatment, cancer survivors should follow the Recommendations for Cancer Prevention.

And, always remember, do not smoke or chew tobacco.

(Reproduced from the 2007 World Cancer Research Fund/ American Institute for Cancer Research report *Food, Nutrition, Physical Activity, and the Prevention of Cancer: a Global Perspective.* www.wcrf.org and www.aicr.org)

In addition, the authors put together a chart illustrating the strength of causal evidence (decreased or increased risk) of related parameters to specific cancers (see Plate 3). It should be stressed that the first two recommendations, although related, are different. You can be lean but you can still be a 'couch potato'. The first recommendation relates to the degree of body fat. It is linked to weight gain and obesity. Excess energy from food is stored as fat. The amount and location of fat varies greatly between people. There is convincing scientific evidence that greater body fatness is a cause of cancer of the esophagus, pancreas, colorectum, breast (postmenopausal), endometrium, and kidney. Body fatness may cause cancer by stimulating an inflammatory response and/or by increasing the amounts of sex steroid hormones and growth factors. Fat is the main source of estrogen synthesis in men and postmenopausal women. Chronic inflammation and increased circulating estrogens can promote cancer development. Recommendation 3 in the list above is designed to control weight gain. Instead of sugary drinks, water or tea may be substitued to help achieve this recommendation. The report states that maintenance of a healthy weight throughout life may be one of the *most important ways* to protect against cancer.

Until the 1960s, physical activity was part of life but recent urbanization and industrialization has caused a sharp decrease in physical activity and has created a sedentary lifestyle. Recommendation 2 is aimed at modern societies. Machines carry out much of the manual labor of yesterday at home and work, cars and public transport have replaced walking and cycling, and outdoor recreation has been replaced by the television and computer. The report recommends moderate physical activity (equivalent to brisk walking) for at least 30 minutes every day, rising ideally to 60 minutes of moderate exercise per day or 30 minutes of vigorous activity per day. A helpful hint to reach this aim can be to incorporate physical activity into household or transport activities if leisure time is tight. An old pastime that could be revisited is planting a vegetable and fruit garden. The rewards of this activity are many, which can satisfy several of the recommendations listed above. First, a garden demands some physical activity for its maintenance. Second, the harvest of the garden will encourage the eating of fresh fruits and vegetables. And as these will be fresh from the vine, they will provide high-quality nutritional value while omitting negative additives that may be used during processing, such as salt and preservatives. (Note that frozen vegetables also maintain high-quality nutritional value, often without additives.)

Mechanisms of physical activity that are involved in reducing cancer risk extend beyond helping to maintain a healthy weight. Additional and independent effects of physical activity include reducing circulating estrogens and male sex steroid hormones, strengthening the immune system, stimulating defense enzymes, and reducing gut transit time.

Recommendation 7 warns that current salt consumption is too high. Daily intake should be less than 6 grams of salt per day. Some processed foods are high in salt. In countries such as the UK, over 80% of the salt in diets comes from processed foods. Salt was once used as a necessary preservative, but refrigeration, freezing, bottling, and canning are modern methods of preservation that do not require salt, although some canned foods contain high levels of salt. Current evidence suggests that salt and salt-preserved foods are a probable cause of increased risk of stomach cancer.

Recommendation 5 states that the intake of red meat (beef, lamb, pork, goat) should be limited and that processed meat should be avoided. Meats are energy-dense foods and can contribute to weight gain. Carcinogens, such as nitrosamines, can form in the body during digestion or while cooking at high temperatures (discussed in Chapter 3). Since meat can be a valuable source of nutrients, such as iron, zinc, and vitamin B12, a recommendation to those who eat red meat is to consume less than 18 oz (500 g) (as eaten) a week. The American Institute for Cancer Research suggests using visual cues to help guide your intake: in general, 3 oz of cooked meat (approximate limit per day) is equivalent to the size of a deck of cards. Processed meats are meats preserved by smoking, curing, salting, or the addition of chemical preservatives. They include hot dogs, sausage, pepperoni, bacon, and ham. There is convincing evidence that processed meats cause colon cancer and probable evidence for contributing to the risk of other cancers.

General advice calls for people to get their nutritional needs from food rather than pills. In the fast pace of modern society where time for food shopping and cooking is limited, some people can be easily tempted to rely on supplements, extra sources of dietary components taken in addition to food. This is not advised because the complexity of whole food components has not yet been untangled fully. Recommendation 8 states that dietary supplements are not recommended for cancer prevention. Let's take the β-Carotene and Retinol Efficacy Trial (CARET) trial as an example. Epidemiological studies showed that people who had diets rich in beta- (or β-) carotene had a reduced risk of lung cancer. Animal studies supported this hypothesis. But when scientists studied the effects of β-carotene supplements on smokers, they were shocked to find that the supplements caused an *increased* risk of cancer. Several explanations may be considered: it may be that a different component of β-carotene-rich foods is responsible for the reduced risk seen in epidemiological studies and/or that β-carotene needs other components present in whole foods to have this effect. This has been an important lesson in the complexity of food and the isolation of components for desired effects. Vitamin and nutritional supplements are often offered in doses that raise body levels to 10–20 times normal physiological levels [note: most do not fall under US Food and Drug Administration (FDA) regulation]. In these cases, a dietary constituent is being used as a drug! More is not necessarily better and, in fact, can be harmful. For now, 'real' whole foods are 'in'.

PLANT FOODS: FRUITS, VEGETABLES, WHOLEGRAINS, AND PULSES

Recommendation 4 listed above states that we should eat a diet rich in a variety of plant foods, including fruits, vegetables, wholegrains, and pulses. Diets rich in plant foods are high in fiber, lower in energy, and help to maintain a healthy weight. The advice to eat five portions of fruits and vegetables a day has been well publicized. Most people are aware that it is healthy to do so. Plate 6 illustrates that there is probable evidence for a decreased risk of many cancers in association with eating fruits and vegetables. As mentioned in Chapter 3, we have a natural defense system against carcinogens. We are just beginning to unravel the importance and potency of components in plant foods that boost our cancer defense systems. Plants contain components called phytochemicals that have evolved to protect them from the harmful effects of the sun. These chemicals in plant foods also protect humans from carcinogens.

Fruits and vegetables are rich in antioxidants. Carcinogens and oxygen metabolism produce products called reactive oxygen species (oxygen free radicals). These are highly reactive forms of oxygen that can react with molecules in our cells, including DNA, and can cause mutations. Remember, mutations are a cause of cancer. Many antioxidants act as a sponge and can chemically 'soak up' free radicals, helping to prevent their negative effects. Both vitamin C and vitamin E act in this manner. Garlic and onions contain organosulfur compounds that are antioxidants.

Another more astonishing mechanism of fruits and vegetables is that some components can actually turn genes on and off! This is quite a finding. Previously we knew about a few select nutrients such as vitamin A and vitamin D that exert their effects via cellular receptors similar to steroid hormone receptors that could turn genes on or off. More recently, new cell pathways have been identified which are triggered by components of foods. These signals are passed through the cell to nuclear transcription factors, similar to growth signals. Interestingly, the genes that are turned on or off by some constituents of fruits and vegetables help guard us against carcinogens.

Broccoli contains a chemical called sulforophane that does just this. It enters cells and stimulates a cell pathway that ultimately turns on genes that produce Phase II enzymes. Phase II enzymes aid in getting rid of some carcinogens by making them more water-soluble for excretion. Thus, by regularly eating these components we are defending ourselves against carcinogens. What a powerful way to protect against cancer.

Is there any evidence that fruits and vegetables protect us from DNA damage? Yes, there is some. DNA damage in blood samples was monitored before, during, and after healthy men consumed a cocktail of fruit juices (330 ml per day over two 2-week periods). Significantly lower levels of DNA damage were observed over the last treatment. The result was not permanent and returned to baseline levels when tested 11 weeks after the experiment ended. So, this provides molecular evidence that daily intake of fruits and vegetables helps protect DNA from mutations.

In my personal opinion, these early indications that food can affect the activity of genes whose products are protective against carcinogens are a landmark in cancer prevention. Its significance is similar to that of the evidence needed to show that smoking causes cancer. Eating well can protect against cancer and we are starting to understand exactly how.

A strategy for meeting the target of five fruits and vegetables a day is easy to achieve once people are aware of its importance. Here are two suggestions.

1. Squeeze a few more vegetables into your meals. It is time for the 'meat-centric' meal to be pushed aside for a plate full of color and texture. Use portobello mushrooms or

eggplant (aubergine) as meat substitutes. Try to limit your portion of red meat in a meal to the size of a deck of cards. Try to have a few meat-free dinners per week, such as a vegetable chilli.

2. Choose fruits and vegetables as snacks: substitute nuts and seeds for potato chips (potato crisps); substitute a fruit smoothie or vegetable soup for a cup of coffee; dip into hummus or salsa; and, for convenience, grab a banana or an apple if you are on the run.

For those who dislike the bitterness of some dark green vegetables, hope is on the way. Chemicals that block bitter receptors on the tongue have recently been patented and approved. Two examples are adenosine monophosphate and GIV3727. Just as salt, artificial sweeteners, and monosodium glutamate are added to foods, soon bitter blockers will be available to help make bitter foods more palatable.

MORE EVIDENCE TO COME

Of course, over time, as methods of research become more powerful and as evidence accumulates, recommendations will be modified. There are several topics on the horizon worth highlighting below.

The first is the link between vitamin D deficiencies and cancer. Low vitamin D level is a public health issue in many places in the world, especially in northern latitudes. Since there is a limited source of vitamin D in many diets, exposure to the sun is needed to synthesize 90–95% of our vitamin D requirement. Exposure to sun may be sparse in some northern locations and lead to inadequate levels. One may speculate that a possible link between physical activity and cancer prevention may include that many physical activities occur outdoors and facilitate sun exposure and the making of vitamin D. The use of sunscreens, though important for protection against skin cancer, may be another factor that limits vitamin D levels. Vitamin D acts like a hormone. Once inside the cell it attaches to and activates the vitamin D receptor. Once activated, this receptor travels into the nucleus of a cell and turns on specific genes. Some of these genes help repair DNA damage, an important mechanism for blocking tumor formation. The report *Food, Nutrition, Physical Activity, and the Prevention of Cancer* states that there is limited suggestive evidence for a link between vitamin D and decreased risk of colon cancer. At present, large clinical trials that examine vitamin D levels and cancer risk are needed. If the results of clinical trials support this link then such evidence could be used to guide policies for vitamin D fortification in particular countries, such as the UK, a land of relatively little sun and few policies for vitamin D fortification.

Another topic on the horizon is tumor cell metabolism. Cell metabolism is the sum of the biochemical pathways that cells use to extract energy from food. It is well known that tumor cells have a metabolism that is very different to that of healthy cells. Tumor metabolism permits rapid cell growth. An increase in glucose metabolism is one distinguishing characteristic of many tumor cells. The increased uptake of fluorescently labeled glucose is a characteristic that allows the detection of tumors during a positron emission tomography (PET) scan.

Knowledge about tumor metabolism is leading to the development of new drugs and even suggestions that specific diets may be beneficial during treatment. Normal cells generate energy by two metabolic pathways: glycolysis, which does not require oxygen, and aerobic pathways that do require oxygen and occur (partly) in mitochondria. There is a shift away from aerobic pathways in cancer, even when oxygen supply is adequate (known as the War-burg effect). Developing treatments that shift metabolism back to aerobic pathways are being investigated as a strategy for cancer management. Future large clinical trials will inform us whether this approach can be successful.

THE GOOD NEWS

The good news is that some cancers can be *prevented* by changes in diet and physical activity. In fact, a third of the most common cancers can be prevented by eating a healthy diet, being physically active, and maintaining a healthy weight. Thanks to the efforts of the World Cancer Research Fund and the American Institute for Cancer Research we have the guidance of evidence-based recom-mendations in the report *Food, Nutrition, Physical Activity, and the Prevention of Cancer: a Global Perspective* to follow. Our understanding of nutrition will allow us to make dietary choices that will reduce the chances of getting cancer. The eating of healthy food should be flaunted and embraced by all. Our lifestyle needs to integrate phys-ical activity. These practices are relatively easy (and fun) to adopt into our daily lives when we truly understand their value. They are as important to the prevention of cancer as not smoking.

8

A FAIRY TALE: FINDING THE CURE TO LEUKEMIA

In the 21st century, there will be patients alive, surviving, and
thriving despite a diagnosis of cancer.

*Brian Druker, MD, Director, Oregon Health and Science
University Knight Cancer Institute, and JELD-WEN
Chair of Leukemia Research*

T his chapter tells the story of how scientists produced a cancer
drug that had a monumental impact on the strategies used for
designing future cancer treatments. The drug is called Gleevec in the
USA and Glivec in Europe and elsewhere. Its generic name is imat-
inib, and it is manufactured by Novartis Pharmaceuticals. It was one
of the first drugs developed to target a specific molecular defect of a
particular cancer. The science behind the making of the drug is what
my former mentor, Professsor Sid Strickland, called 'three little pig
science'; it was science built not of straw, nor sticks, but of bricks. The
science followed a solid logical sequence over decades of research:
first identify the defect in the disease, then understand the mechanism
of how it causes the disease, and lastly figure out how to block its

action. The development of Gleevec has unfolded like a fairy tale with a happy ending. And the story has some special heroes.

Chronic myelogenous leukemia (CML) is a type of leukemia (a cancer of the blood) that makes up about a fifth of all leukemias. The annual incidence is one or two cases per 100,000 people per year, which translates into about 800 new cases each year in the UK and 5000 new cases each year in the USA. Before the year 2000 prognosis for patients was grim. The disease progressed through different stages to become fatal within 4–6 years. The early phase of the disease is called the chronic phase (lasting 3–5 years). This phase is followed by the accelerated phase (lasting 3–9 months) and blast crisis (lasting 3–6 months). Treatment available at the time, alpha- (or α-) interferon, often had uncomfortable side-effects such as flu-like symptoms and nausea. Inconveniently, α-interferon needs to be injected under the skin every day. Hope for a bone marrow transplant, the only proven cure, was often far away beyond many obstacles, such as finding a matching donor and being fit enough to undergo the procedure.

Bone marrow transplantation is an amazing treatment when it can be performed. It was the first demonstration of a stem cell therapy. The bone marrow is the place where blood (hematopoietic) stem cells reside. These stem cells have the ability to perpetuate themselves and generate all the mature blood cell types simultaneously. That is, when a stem cell divides to form two daughter cells, one of the daughter cells is a stem cell and the other becomes more specialized towards becoming a specific blood cell type (such as a white blood cell or red blood cell). As a strategy for treatment of leukemia, the patient's bone marrow is irradiated to kill the leukemic blood cells and is replaced by a donor's marrow which is able to repopulate the patient with stem cells needed to continually produce healthy blood cells. A 'match' is needed to prevent immunological rejection by the recipient.

The first step towards finding a treatment for any disease is to identify the defect of the disease. Scientists asked the question, 'what is the difference between a normal blood cell and a leukemic blood cell?' The molecular defect of CML was revealed by careful observation of leukemic cells. Indeed, the defect, a shortened chromosome, was able to be 'seen' under a microscope (Figure 16). It was the first chromosome abnormality to be associated with a cancer. Unfortunately, this is a characteristic that is not very common for other cancers. The shortened chromosome was named after the city in which it was identified: the Philadelphia chromosome.

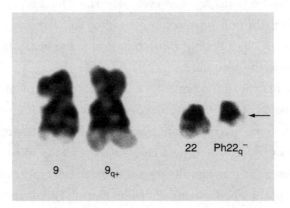

FIG 16 Light micrograph of two chromosome pairs including the chromosomal translocation that causes chronic myelogenous leukemia (CML). From left is a normal chromosome 9, a larger defective chromosome 9_q+, a normal chromosome 22, and a smaller defective chromosome, the Philadelphia chromosome, Ph22q$^-$, which carries the bcr_ahl fusion gene indicated by the arrow.

The Philadelphia chromosome is the result of a repair gone wrong: two chromosomes break and are joined to their wrong halves during repair. (You may remember from Chapter 3 that exposure to ionizing radiation is carcinogenic because it can cause DNA double-stranded breaks and chromosomal translocations.) The Philadelphia chromosome is made up of part of chromosome 22 and part of chromosome 9. The genes at the joint of the repair of the DNA breaks are altered. The new chromosomal construction brings together the *bcr* gene and the *abl* gene and forms a *bcr-abl* fusion gene (Figure 16).

Could it be that the Philadelphia chromosome makes a normal blood cell turn into a cancer cell? In other words, was this truly the defect that causes cancer rather than just a feature of this cancer? To answer this question, G.Q. Daley, R.A. Van Etten, and D. Baltimore at the Massachusetts Institute of Technology determined whether they could cause leukemia in healthy animals by introducing the *bcr-abl* fusion gene into their bone marrow, where blood cells are produced. They did this via bone marrow transplantation. Cells from marrow were isolated from the long bones of young mice and viruses were used to carry the fusion gene into these cells. Infected marrow was transplanted back into mice that had had their existing marrow destroyed by irradiation. After several months of waiting, examination of the experimental mice revealed symptoms very similar to patients with CML: high white-blood-cell count and enlargement of the spleen. This evidence, published in 1990, confirmed that the *bcr-abl* gene alone could cause leukemia.

The second step is to learn *how* the defect causes the disease. In healthy cells, the product of the *abl* gene, a tyrosine kinase (see Chapter 5 for a discussion about kinases), modifies many other proteins in the nucleus when needed for cell growth. Because of the new association formed by the chromosomal translocation of the Philadelphia chromosome, the *abl* gene loses its normal regulation and the activity of its product, the ABL protein, is stuck in the 'on' position. That is, its kinase activity cannot be switched off. Furthermore, it is relocated to the cytoplasm of the cell instead of its normal location, the nucleus. The product from the fusion gene is not only unregulated but it is in the wrong place within the cell. We know that the kinase activity is necessary for causing cancer because when the scientists blocked the kinase activity of the fusion protein by introducing mutations into the fusion gene, the triggering of cancer did not occur. As a consequence of this constitutive ('always on') kinase activity, white blood cells undergo uncontrolled growth, a characteristic of leukemia.

The final step towards finding a treatment is to find something that will block the action of the defect. The knowledge about the mechanism working via a kinase gave the scientists an idea. They reasoned that if they could make a drug that could stop the kinase activity of this protein that is stuck in the 'on' position, they may be able to treat the disease. Scientists from a Switzerland-based company, now called Novartis, searched a collection of chemicals using a strategy called screening. This strategy is like adding ingredients from the kitchen shelf, one at a time, on to some test cells and looking to see which one works. Their efforts pointed to a likely candidate that could block kinase activity. Small chemical changes were made by chemists to modify the candidate drug for better drug-like qualities and improved specificity. For example, a methyl group was added here to improve specificity and an

N-methyl piperazine was added there to make the drug more soluble and able to be taken orally (a drug that could be taken orally instead of by daily injection would improve the quality of life of CML patients). Finally, Gleevec was created. After testing the drug in cell culture and animal cells, scientists began clinical trials to test the drug in humans.

The fairy tale story of Gleevec told in this chapter has many heroes: far too many to name them all as the work described here condenses 50 years of science. However, I would like to profile one man who made great contributions to the field. His name is Brian J. Druker. Druker started his biological training at the University of California, San Diego. After tasting molecular biology as an undergraduate, Druker continued to Medical School. Quickly he blended the two subjects and wrote in his dissertation that only through a molecular understanding of cancer would we be able to treat cancer rationally. His internships and residency found him caring for leukemia patients. Little would his patients of that time know of the great advances Druker would make for their disease. Druker continued to study the molecular biology of cancer and he made a career decision to study kinases in leukemia. At the time there were two schools of thought about kinases: one school saw the importance of kinases in disease and the potential for them to be drug targets; the other school comprised the skeptics. Although it may be difficult to believe today, Druker was told that he had no future. However, the obstacles and setbacks were only temporary and Druker found himself in a fresh and encouraging environment at the Oregon Health and Science University. From here he, and colleagues from Novartis, tested Gleevec and began clinical trials that changed the course of cancer treatment.

All drugs must be tested in a stepwise fashion in clinical trials before they can be approved for public use. The testing that occurred before this stage was done using cell culture, test tubes, and animal models (mice). Taking a new drug for use in humans is a huge leap and must be done with care. Phase I trials examine a range of drug doses for safety in a small number of patients (20–100). The results from the first trials for Gleevec were almost too good to be true. Patients showed a good response (it worked!) and there were minimal side-effects. Surprisingly, the good response worried some of the scientists working on the drug because they thought that most known effective cancer drugs are very toxic and have severe side-effects. They thought that since this new drug was not toxic it probably would not hold up in later and larger Phase II trials. But they were wrong. The drug worked so well in Phase II trials on a larger number of patients that it was approved in record time, in May 2001, just three years after the start of the Phase I study. It was the fastest-approved cancer drug in history. Druker commented on the three-year period from the first clinical trial to US Food and Drug Administration (FDA) approval: '…when you think about it, that's truly remarkable. The average drug approval time is between five and seven years. We did it in three.'

The scientists asked the question, 'is the drug working the way we think it is working?' That is, they had designed the drug to block a specific kinase activity and now wanted to examine whether blocking this molecular activity was the reason the drug was successful. This was fairly easy to test. Since kinases add small chemicals called phosphate groups to target proteins, they were able to see whether normal ABL targets were modified with phosphate groups after treatment with Gleevec. In this way, they demonstrated that Gleevec blocks tyrosine kinase activity in CML. The Gleevec story is an example of translational research; that is, research that ushers the movement from bench to bedside, from laboratory to clinic. Translational research is all about knowing your target and the ABL kinase proved to be perfect for the discovery of a successful drug.

THE GOOD NEWS

The good news is that now people with CML have a better prognosis with Gleevec, a drug with a 98% *response rate* in early-stage patients. So, patients with a diagnosis of CML have a five-year survival rate of 95% rather than a death sentence (previously, median survival was three to five years).

The story gets even better: the same drug targets two other receptor kinases (c-kit and PDGFR), which play a role in a type of stomach/intestinal cancer called gastrointestinal stromal cancer (or GIST) and in the brain cancer glioblastoma, respectively. The knowledge that 90% of GIST patients have mutations that cause the kit kinase receptor to be 'always on' suggested that GIST might be treatable by Gleevec. Gleevec was approved for treatment of GIST and so this drug will touch the lives of the 5000–6000 new patients diagnosed with GIST each year in the USA. Noteworthy is that GIST is unresponsive to chemotherapies and radiotherapies. Surgery was the main form of treatment, although recurrence was common. Gleevec is being tested in clinical trials for the treatment of glioblastoma.

The most important consequence of the science behind Gleevec was that a new path was laid down for the discovery of new targeted therapies for cancer. It is important to note that Gleevec was the first tyrosine kinase inhibitor to be used as a cancer therapy. As stated above, many in the field were skeptical about whether kinases could serve as a cancer drug target because there are many kinases in the cell and all kinases have similar active sites because they do the same thing: they add phosphate groups to proteins. But drugs have been identified that are able to act selectively only against a few particular kinases. Many other successful cancer treatments that work as tyrosine kinase inhibitors have followed. The list includes Iressa (gefitinib; AstraZeneca), Nexavar (sorafenib; Bayer Pharm), Tarceva (erlotinib; Genentech), and Tykerb (lapatinib; GlaxoSmithKline). New targeted therapies promise fewer side-effects than conventional therapies. Many conventional therapies target DNA non-specifically and as a result affect healthy cells as well as cancer cells.

The not so good news is that Gleevec does not work for all patients and those with advanced disease often relapse one year later because their cells become drug-resistant. But, scientists have figured out how drug resistance occurs. In many cases, it is because cancer cells acquire additional mutations, some of which interfere with the physical binding of Gleevec to the kinase. This scenario is not too dissimilar from the rise of antibiotic-resistant strains of bacteria. Methods that allowed scientists to visualize the structure of the ABL kinase protein when bound to Gleevec revealed structural changes in drug-resistant mutant forms of the kinase. Although 50 different mutations that interfere with Gleevec binding have been identified, only six account for 60–70% of all mutations. Second-generation kinase inhibitors are drugs that can inhibit some *abl* mutants that are resistant against Gleevec.

Dasatinib is an example of a second-generation kinase inhibitor approved by the FDA and European Medicines Agency to treat Gleevec-resistant CML. Dasatinib can inhibit five out of the six most common mutations. It is possible that a second mutation may lead to dasatinib resistance and so combinations of inhibitors are being examined to prevent additional drug resistance.

9

CANCER SCREENING WORKS!

Cancer mortality in both screening trials and in service screening programmes indicates a substantial saving of lives from breast, cervical, and bowel cancer. Screening clearly saves lives.

Stephen W. Duffy, Professor of Cancer Screening, Wolfson Institute of Preventive Medicine, Barts and the London School of Medicine and Dentistry, Queen Mary University of London

Cancer screening is all about spotting cancer *before* symptoms appear. This is an ambitious goal since most diseases are recognized by the appearance of symptoms. Cancer screening involves testing whole populations for structural, biochemical, or cellular changes that expose the early developmental stages of cancer. Cancer is a disease that is characterized by the ability to spread to other parts of the body and this feature is the most difficult aspect to treat. It is a fact that catching cancer early, preferably before spreading, is important for a patient's long-term outcome (prognosis). Cancer screening may not only improve prognosis and reduce cancer deaths, but it may also allow for less aggressive treatments.

Some screening tests not only detect early cancers but even identify *precancerous* changes and these tests aim to *prevent* cancer. We have learned enough about the process of carcinogenesis to be able to recognize changes in normal cell growth that indicate a potential to become cancerous. Medical tests may include imaging techniques such as X-rays and techniques that examine individual cells and/or molecules, such as DNA.

Public health campaigns have made us aware of screening for breast cancer, cervical cancer, and colon cancer. Research is ongoing to extend the list of tests for screening other cancers. The USA, the UK, and Australia prepare numerous publications and web pages that report on current cancer screening guidelines (see the Bibliography listing for Chapter 9 at the end of the book).

BREAST CANCER SCREENING

Let's begin our discussion by examining the use of mammography for breast cancer screening. Mammography is the use of X-rays to detect tumors in the breast of women who do not have any symptoms of breast cancer. The American Cancer Society recommends annual mammography for women who are 40 years and older. In the UK breast screening is recommended every three years for all women who are 50 years and older. Many other countries in Europe, such as France, Finland, Italy, and the Netherlands, as well as Australia, recommend mammography screening from age 50 years whereas Japan recommends screening from the age of 40. Mammography is less effective in younger women who are premenopausal because the breast is denser and tumors are more difficult to see. After menopause, the breast becomes mainly composed of fat and is less dense, making tumors more visible. In 2009 the US Preventative Service Task Force presented an analysis of screening that also took harmful effects such as false-positive results into account and recommended against mammography screening for women under 50 years. Controversy exists for using mammography on women younger than 50 years.

The UK National Health Service (NHS) Breast Screening Program was started in 1988, is government funded, and provides a free service for women within the defined age group (currently 50–70 years but this range is due to be extended to 47–73 years by 2012). The screening program offered by the UK is commendable due to its proactive outreach approach. Women receive a personal letter upon reaching 50 years, inviting them for their first screen. Letters of recall are sent every three years. About 1.7 million women are screened each year in the UK. This equates to an acceptance level of about 74% in those aged 50 year and older. This may be compared to the USA, where about 67% of women 40 years and older reported having a mammogram within the past two years. A participation rate of only 57% has been reported for Australia's BreastScreen Program. Although the Japanese government has recommended mammography screening since 2000, the participation rate in Japan is under 5%. This figure underscores the lack of effectiveness of screening policies after transfer of cancer screening responsibilities from national to local government in 1998. Smaller average breast size in Japanese women (compared to average breast size in Western women) has caused technical challenges in screening equipment and modifications are needed. Breast cancer incidence peaks at age 40–49 years in Japan compared to a peak at 70–79 years in Western countries and so compliance to

Extended figure legends are described in the List of plates on p.xvii

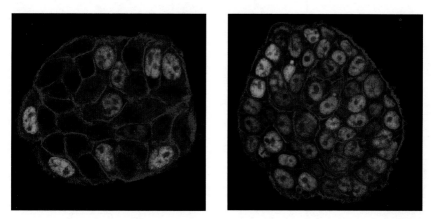

Plate 1

P53 becomes active in cells after UV treatment.

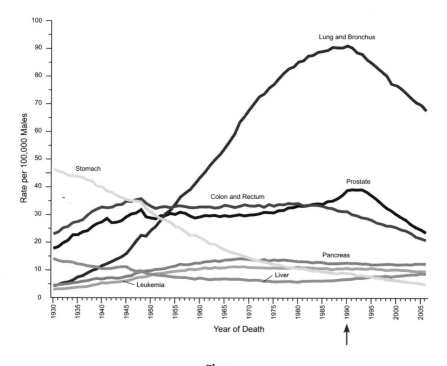

Plate 2

Annual age-adjusted cancer death rates among males for selected cancers in the USA, 1930–2006.

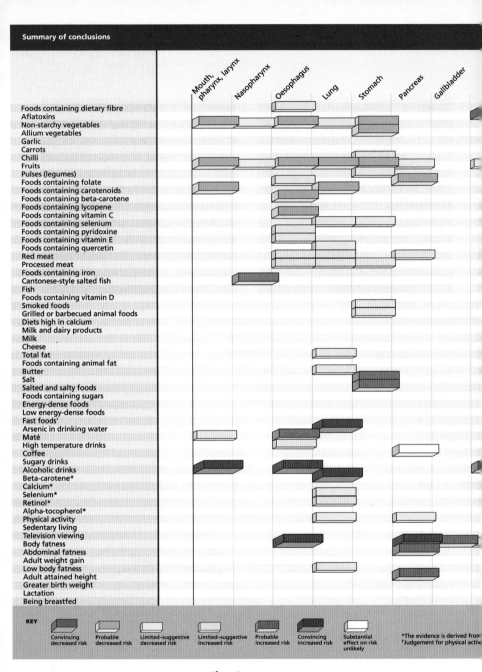

Plate 3
Strength of the evidence causally relating food, nutrition,
and physical activity to the risk of cancer.

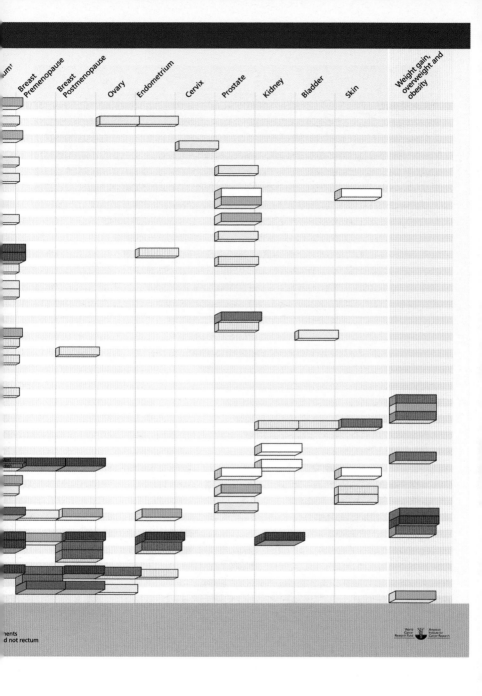

ments
d not rectum

World Cancer Research Fund   American Institute for Cancer Research

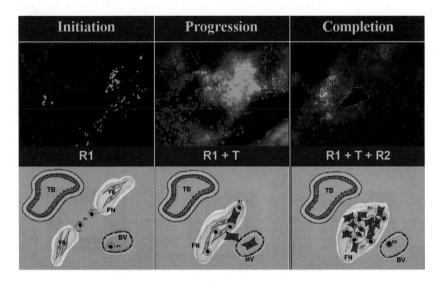

Plate 4
Evidence of the premetastatic niche.

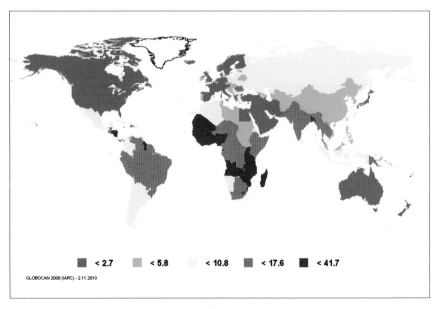

Plate 5
Estimated age-standardized mortality rate per 100,000 for cervix uteri, all ages.

screening early in life is of great importance. These observations shout out for rapid improvements in Japan.

Women with breast implants should undergo routine mammography screening. Since implants may block radiation, radiographers may need some extra time to take additional X-rays and/or adjust the positioning of the X-rays. And so it is good practice to state you have implants when making an appointment for mammography.

Some people are affected by an hereditary breast cancer syndrome whereby they have inherited not breast cancer itself, but an increased *risk* of breast cancer. About 5% of all cases of breast cancer are due to an inherited predisposition. High-risk patients include those with inherited mutations in the *BRCA1* or *BRCA2* genes. The *BRCA1* and *BRCA2* genes code for proteins that play a role in the regulation of gene expression and DNA repair, so cells from these patients are vulnerable to mutation. Affected patients should be screened more vigorously. The American Cancer Society recommends that women at high risk should get a mammogram and magnetic resonance imaging (MRI) scan every year and that women with *BRCA* gene mutations should begin this screening at age 25.

Some inconveniences and disadvantages exist with mammography screening. Although not invasive, nobody particularly enjoys going to the doctor to get their breasts squeezed between two cold metal plates and zapped by radiation. Although low-dose radiation is used (much lower and more controlled compared to the 1970s), one may note that radiation is a carcinogen. A positive result from a mammogram is not a diagnosis. It directs you to undergo further tests, such as a biopsy for a diagnosis. The occurrence of false-positive results may be another disadvantage of screening. You may have a positive result from a mammogram that leads you to have a biopsy which then turns out to be negative. Although relieved at hearing that the biopsy is negative you would have gone through a stressful time and an unnecessary invasive procedure. Another disadvantage is over-diagnosis. This refers to finding an abnormal growth or even a small tumor that would not have led to cancer. It is known that some small tumors lie dormant and do not become cancerous. Over-diagnosis is becoming more of an issue as screening tests become more sensitive. We await better markers to distinguish between dangerous and less-dangerous abnormal growths. But since 1 million people get breast cancer each year, the inconveniences and disadvantages are outweighed by the potential consequences of not being screened. Currently, 61% of breast cancers are diagnosed at a localized stage, for which the five-year survival rate is 98%!

The experience of getting a positive result upon a routine screening visit is still shocking to most people. The events that follow create sensations like being on a rollercoaster. First there is the anxiety of going for a biopsy with feelings that fluctuate between 'this is the end' and 'it must be a false alarm'. The biopsy is carried out, leaving you feeling bruised and vulnerable. You wait helplessly for the verdict. The verdict is positive. Those same conflicted feelings that you had upon hearing the positive screening results reappear but are greatly intensified. This is the climb and fall of the rollercoaster that leaves you screaming. And then, you numbingly give yourself up to the healthcare system. Generally, you are in good hands. The doctors give you an abundance of statistics and information, more than you can consume. You may have decisions to make about surgery: lumpectomy versus mastectomy. You are scheduled for your first round of radiation and surprisingly, after treatment, you don't feel as bad as you had imagined. Yes, you do feel tired but at the same time you find a new strength in living. You give permission for further tests to be done that will provide more information regarding the strategy for your future treatment. You find yourself lucky as the results suggest that you will not need chemotherapy. You begin taking anti-estrogen medication that, reassuringly, has been in use for several decades. Periodic check-ups will be your future but the words 'all-clear' leave you with thoughts of living your life. Of course and unfortunately, this scenario is not the case for everyone. But now, at least, stories with this type of ending happen more often than in the past.

The good news is that mammography screening saves lives. Many studies have evaluated the effectiveness of screening, although not all previous studies reported a benefit. Some controversy existed for a short period of time after Danish investigators (Gøtzsche and Nielsen, 2011) claimed that many of the studies that reported benefit were flawed. But this was resolved by a group of 24 experts from 11 countries who were commissioned by the International Agency for Cancer Research of the World Health Organization. In 2002, this group re-examined data from previous trials and concluded that mammography screening is beneficial for women between 50 and 69 years. From this evaluation it is estimated that the reduction in mortality from breast cancer due to screening is about 35%. This translates to saving 1400 lives per year in the UK. A similar success was reported for Australia in that there was a 21–28% reduction in mortality in the 50–69-year age group due to the national BreastScreen Programme.

CERVICAL CANCER SCREENING

Cervical cancer screening is another important health issue for women. This type of screening detects abnormal cells and can catch precancerous growth. The Pap test (or Pap smear) is routinely done in a doctor's office or clinic. A small spatula or cervical brush is used to take a sample of cells from the cervix. The sample is spread onto a microscope slide creating a smear of cells, washed in a preservative, and analyzed in a laboratory. The current guidelines from the National Cancer Institute (USA) and the NHS (UK) recommend screening once every three years. In the UK, similar to the breast screening program, women receive an invitation in the mail, every three years. Australia's cervical cancer screening program recommends Pap smears every 2 years from age 18 to 69. To give one a sense of numbers, in England, in 2007–2008, 3.2 million women (aged 25–64) were screened. If the tests are abnormal, patients may undergo fairly simple treatment to remove abnormal cells. The treatment options include laser therapy, cryotherapy (freezing), or electrosurgical procedures.

Again, the consequences of screening are beneficial. About 75% of cervical cancer cases are prevented in women who are screened routinely (Cancer Research UK, National Cancer Institute). A historical perspective reveals our progress over time. As late as the 1940s, cervical cancer was a major cause of death in women of childbearing years in the USA. The introduction of only one test in the 1950s, the Pap test, led to a 74% decrease in the incidence of cervical cancer from 1955 to 1992. In the USA cervical cancer has moved from being one of the most common cancers in women to ranking 14th. Unfortunately there are places in the world where screening is not easily available or affordable. The worldwide cervical cancer burden is heavy, as it is the third most frequent cause of cancer death, accounting for 300,000 deaths per year. The good news is that cervical cancer screening works, but we need to extend the practice worldwide.

Technically, there is some room for improvement. Variations in technique and human error can sometimes cause damage to the cells when the sample is applied to the microscope slide and as a result false-positive readings may result. That is, abnormal cells may be detected because of mishandling of the sample instead of being a true representation of cells within the patient. So, a newer method of handling samples, called a liquid-based Pap test, has been developed whereby collected cells are removed from the instrument by rinsing them in liquid preservative and slides are prepared, not by human hands, but by an automated device in a laboratory. In addition, computer-automated readers are being used to read the Pap slides to reduce human error in reading samples.

Although we welcome the introduction of a new cervical cancer vaccine (discussed in Chapter 12) which protects against 70% of cervical cancers, cervical screening needs to be maintained to prevent cancer in the 30% who cannot be protected by the vaccine. It is crucial not to create a false sense of security in thinking that the vaccine will completely abolish cervical cancer. This is a point that needs to be emphasized again and again, so as not to undo our progress in reducing cervical cancer incidence.

COLORECTAL CANCER SCREENING

Screening for colorectal cancer is one of the more recent screening programs to have been introduced. Let's begin with some facts and numbers. Colorectal cancer is the third leading cause of cancer death in the USA in both men and women. This translates into about 50,000 deaths per year. The importance of screening becomes obvious as one learns that when colorectal cancer is found early and treated, the five-year relative survival rate is 90%. And screening not only detects early disease but it also spots precancerous polyps that, when removed, can prevent the disease. Yes, colorectal cancer, the third leading killer, can actually be prevented through screening!

In the USA the American Cancer Society recommends several options for screening beginning at age 50. It states that the first four tests shown below are preferred because they can find precancerous growths called polyps as well as cancer, although they are more invasive:

flexible sigmoidoscopy every five years,

colonoscopy every 10 years,

double-contrast barium enema every five years,

CT colonoscopy (virtual colonoscopy) every five years,

fecal occult blood test every year,

fecal immunochemical test every year,

stool DNA (sDNA) test, uncertain interval.

Europe falls behind in offering such a comprehensive colorectal cancer screening program. In the UK the NHS Bowel Screening Program invites men and women aged 60–69 years to take a fecal occult blood test using a home kit. This test detects small amounts of blood that may be released from precancerous polyps and cancer.

(Note that minute bleeding may be intermittent and may be missed at the time of testing.) The home kit involves collecting a sample of stool, applying a smear of stool to a sample card, and mailing the sample card to a laboratory. Australia has a national Bowel Screening Program similar to the UK except that it invites people from age 50 to use a fecal occult blood test from home. Improvements are on the board. UK Prime Minister David Cameron announced that the screening technique called Flexi-Scope (flexible sigmoidoscopy) is to be included in the NHS Bowel Screening Program.

The home test is saving lives for some who take the time to use the kit. Take William for example. Although his friends threw their kit in the garbage, William, who had just turned 60 years old, decided to take the test because he lost both of his parents to cancer and wanted to do all he could to prevent a similar fate. Taking the test proved to be a life-saving decision. Two weeks after sending off his sample card he was contacted and asked to undergo further tests. A cancerous tumor was found and removed by surgery a few weeks later. William said: 'It was such a shock to find out that I had cancer because I had no symptoms at all. I felt brand new....It's odd to think that you can have cancer and not have a clue that you've got it....I dread to think what would have happened had I not done the test as it would have taken some considerable time for me to get symptoms by which time it may have been too late.'

William was fortunate to catch his cancer early. He did not need chemotherapy or radiotherapy. He only needs to undergo regular monitoring. William urges his friends to complete the home test. He explains that it only took five minutes and it was the best thing he ever did.

In the USA screening uptake is only 50% and so there is need for improvement. Let's examine why this figure may be low. First, there are several options available and although this allows some freedom of choice, it may also introduce a level of uncertainty: 'what test?' and 'how often?' Colonoscopy is viewed as the gold standard. It involves tunneling a small video camera on a long tube through the intestine to view the intestinal lining. Colonoscopy may be superior to other tests in several regards, such as its sensitivity; it can detect small precancerous polyps. But it does require a colon-emptying medication and a sedative, and also carries some risks, such as the possibility of making a hole in the colon. More recently we have seen the emergence of non-invasive testing. Colorectal cancer provides clues of its presence by leaving evidence in stool which can be collected in the comfort of your own home. This is the future! Most people would prefer to give up a sample of bodily fluid/waste rather than undergo an invasive technique in a doctor's office or clinic to participate in screening, but the tests must be effective at detecting early cancer and, in the best-case scenario, precancerous changes.

Tests better than the fecal occult blood test are emerging thanks to our better understanding of the molecular biology of tumors. The knowledge of the genetic and epigenetic changes that occur during colorectal cancer progression and the technical advances in recovering DNA from a stool sample have led to the development of screens that analyze stool DNA instead of blood. Genes that are often mutated in colorectal cancer (85%) include the *adenomatous polyposis coli* (APC) gene, the *p53* gene, and the *K-ras* gene. A test that included examining stool DNA for 21 different mutations within these three genes was compared to a fecal occult blood test. The stool DNA test was found to be more sensitive than the fecal occult blood test (Imperiale et al., 2004), but unfortunately it was not as sensitive as colonoscopy. An improved stool DNA test that examines only two markers, hypermethylated vimentin gene (found in 80% of colorectal cancers) and a two-site DNA integrity assay, has been examined more recently. The results show high sensitivity (83%) and high specificity (82%) for colorectal cancer. The simplification of the test makes it easier to run in local laboratories, and the cost is lower as well. I am certain further modifications will be made to improve this type of test and that it will become the gold standard of colon cancer screening in the future.

Screening schedules should be increased for those who are at high risk of getting colorectal cancer due to hereditary predispositions. The most common hereditary colon cancer syndrome is Lynch syndrome (also known as hereditary nonpolyposis colorectal cancer, or HNPCC). Those affected with Lynch syndrome have inherited an *increased risk* of developing a range of cancers including colon cancer, though not all patients will develop cancer. Patients with Lynch syndrome carry a mutation in one of four DNA-repair genes and so their cells are vulnerable to mutations. Heather Hampel, a cancer genetic counselor at Ohio State University, and her colleagues have carried out several large genetic studies of patients with colon cancer. Commenting on the results of these studies, Heather states 'the fact that one in 35 colorectal cancer patients has Lynch syndrome is staggering, and when you consider the implications for other family members, it could be considered a significant public health issue'. Many patients are not aware of their family history for this disease. Family members who do not have the mutation are at normal risk and only need to follow the guidelines mentioned above. Family members who have the mutation but do not yet have cancer should begin screening at a younger age and more frequently (colonoscopy every one or two years beginning at age 25), because the average age of colon cancer diagnosis for these patients is 44 years old. Patients with Lynch syndrome have a 50% chance of passing the disease to their offspring, an observation made by Dr Lynch in 1966. Hampel and her colleagues recommend that all newly diagnosed colorectal cancer patients be screened for Lynch syndrome so that family histories can be accurate and informative.

The introduction of newer and less-intrusive tests, along with education and health insurance coverage, may help improve the number of people undergoing screening. This is an important goal. It has been estimated that appropriate testing could save more than half of those who will die from colorectal cancer.

SCREENING METHODS ON THE HORIZON

The use of non-invasive methods of screening for many cancers will make a significant contribution towards whole-population participation. Saliva, urine, and blood sampling hold biochemical and molecular clues that will allow such screening to take place. Such clues include modified (methylated) and mutated genes and proteins, and are called **biomarkers** (see Table 2). The use of biomarkers is being investigated for oral cancer, lung cancer, ovarian cancer, bladder cancer, and prostate cancer. Many small studies using bodily fluids as screening samples have been carried out but large controlled studies are needed for their validation. Recently it has been reported that a blood test that examines six genes linked

Type of cancer	Source of biomarkers	Candidate biomarkers
Ovarian	Serum markers	CA-125 plus others (e.g. osteopontin)
Liver	Serum markers	Alpha-fetoprotein (AFP), AFP-L3
Lung	Sputum	Mitochondrial mutations, methylation panel
Prostate	Urine	PCA3, methylated genes (e.g. *p16*, *ARF*, *GSTP1*)
Bladder	Urine	Methylated DNA, Aurora A,B,C, mitochondrial DNA alterations

Table 2. Candidate biomarkers. Data from National Cancer Institute, The Early Detection Research Network (2008) *Investing in Translational Research on Biomarkers of Early Cancer and Cancer Risk*, fourth report. http://edrn.nci. nih.gov/docs/progress-reports/edrn_4th-report_200801.pdf.

to prostate cancer may be combined with the conventional prostate-specific antigen (PSA) test to improve the accuracy of cancer detection but this needs to be confirmed in a large controlled study. PSA is a protein produced by prostate gland cells and blood levels can be measured and used to detect disease. Elevated levels can arise in both non-cancerous and cancerous disease and therefore PSA levels alone are not sufficient to diagnose prostate cancer but are useful for indicating the need for further tests.

The expansion of studies will follow our growing understanding of cancer genomics and proteomics. Further in the future is cancer nanotechnology. It also promises to yield improvements in screening, and may be a means for continual biomonitoring. That is, it has been proposed that nanoscale devices may be able to monitor biochemical and molecular changes that occur over time.

THE GOOD NEWS

Screening can detect precancerous changes and early stage cancer. Consequently, some cancers can be prevented or at least treated early to give a better prognosis. Both the UK and the USA have vigorous screening practices in place that are saving lives (Figure 17).

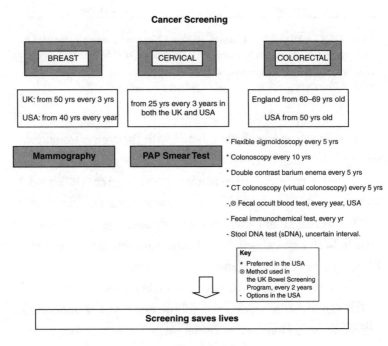

FIG 17 Cancer screening.

10

LET'S TALK ABOUT IT

Scientists are communicating more now than ever before. The
resulting collaborations accelerate the speed of breakthroughs in
cancer research and bring new treatments to patients at a faster pace.
There is never a good time to get cancer; however, those who are
navigating the cancer maze today benefit from many excellent print
and online resources that provide vital information and support.

*Margaret Foti, PhD, MD (hc), Chief Executive Officer, American Association of Cancer
Research*

Cancer has not been easy to talk about in society but major
positive changes have occurred. Progress began with initiatives at the national level, such as those led by the National Cancer
Institute in the USA. The desire to be proactive in communicating cancer awareness spread through philanthropic societies and
celebrity circles. And some amazing initiatives were developed
by motivated individuals and small businesses. The few examples
described below demonstrate both the power of concerted efforts

of thousands of people and also the strength of some energetic individuals.

CANCER INFORMATION SERVICE

The first major contribution to cancer communication came from establishment of the Cancer Information Service (or CIS) by the US National Cancer Institute in 1975 to fulfill new responsibilities for educating the public, patients, and health professionals. Although the National Cancer Act of 1971 began the war on cancer, the personal story of one individual politician, Massachusetts senator Edward M. Kennedy, ignited the public desire for access to best care. The influential Kennedy family was able to secure the most up-to-date information and treatment for Edward Kennedy's son who had been diagnosed with a sarcoma. At the time, the public did not have access to the latest cancer information. The CIS was set up to provide free and easy access to the latest cancer information for all. But this was not an easy task, as you can imagine, because there was a lack of communication technologies in the seventies: no advanced fax machines and no e-mail systems. Marion Morra, one of the early pioneers of the CIS, told me that it is 'funny to think of how primitive it all was': information files were kept on a Rollerdex and it could take a full day to transmit a long document to a specific location using the then state-of-the-art telecopiers. The creation of the toll-free telephone number, 1-800-4-CANCER, by CIS had a big impact for cancer patients and their families. This service, which still serves the American public today, has served over 5 million people. Of course, new technologies have allowed the CIS to provide additional services that now include access to treatment databases, including clinical trials, a publications ordering service, e-mail, and instant messaging. The good practice of the CIS has spread and now there are more than 20 members of the international CIS group across the world. Members of the international CIS group are listed at www.icisg.org/meet_memberslist.htm.

CANCER RESEARCH UK AND THE AMERICAN ASSOCIATION FOR CANCER RESEARCH

The first specialized cancer research organization in the UK was set up in 1902 by the Royal Colleges of Surgeons and Physicians, and since then this organization has evolved into Cancer Research UK, one of the largest charities worldwide. Cancer Research UK supports the work of around 5,000 scientists, doctors, and nurses across the UK, investigating all aspects of cancer. Its major goal is to reduce cancer mortality through research to improve prevention, early diagnosis, and treatment. The charity also provides high-quality information for people affected by cancer, the public, and health professionals. Through its campaigning it aims to influence public policy and to keep cancer at the top of the public health agenda. Recently, Cancer Research UK, along with several partners, launched a program to improve genetic testing services and to collect genetic data on tumors in the UK, paving the way for personalized medicine (discussed in Chapter 13).

In the USA, the American Association for Cancer Research (AACR) was formed in 1907 by only 11 research scientists and clinicians who saw a need for improving cancer research and treatments. The last hundred years have shown tremendous growth with the current membership of 32,000 basic, translational, and clinical researchers, healthcare professionals, cancer survivors, and advocates in the USA and more than 90 other countries. The AACR has been led by Chief Executive Officer Margaret Foti since 1982. In addition to organizing special conferences throughout the year on a wide variety of topics in cancer research, treatment, and patient care, the AACR organizes an Annual Meeting that hosts more than 18,000 attendees from all over the world. I have been an attendee for the last five years and would not think of missing one purely from the standpoint of it being *the* time and place for cancer research information loading. So, for those who have been recently diagnosed with cancer, try not to feel alone but seek comfort in the fact that the people who attend these meetings are dedicating their life to the cause. The president of the AACR in 2010, Professor Tyler Jacks, stated in an interview that the generation of cancer researchers that are emerging will see our ability to control the disease come to fruition.

The AACR has also created the Scientist-Survivor Program that brings patients and survivor advocates together with research scientists. Communication between the two groups allows survivors to receive first-hand scientific information and allows scientists to understand the issues affecting cancer survivors. The ACCR also publishes vast numbers of research papers in its journals and policy statements, such as the policy statement on Tobacco and Cancer (2010). Here the AACR identified policy and research initiatives critical for overcoming the full spectrum of the tobacco problem. In addition to calling for evidence-based strategies, it also urges the USA to ratify the World Health Organization Framework

Convention on Tobacco Control, a treaty that aims to tackle the problems of tobacco use globally.

PINK RIBBONS AND BREAST CANCER AWARENESS

The most widely recognized symbol of breast cancer awareness is the pink ribbon. New York philanthropist and business woman Evelyn H. Lauder has made huge contributions to breast cancer awareness and research. In 1992, Evelyn, daughter-in-law of Estée Lauder, along with Alexandra Penny, former Editor of *SELF* magazine, co-created the pink ribbon as a symbol of breast health. Since 1992, the Estée Lauder Companies' Breast Cancer Awareness (BCA) campaign has given away more than 100 million pink ribbons and millions of informational brochures at its cosmetic counters around the world. The pink ribbon is one of the most successful marketing campaigns ever launched and has become the ubiquitous symbol for breast health. In 2000 the BCA broadened its 'Pink' awareness campaign and began illuminating historic landmarks such as the Empire State Building, Niagara Falls, the Tower of London, the Leaning Tower of Pisa, and the Tokyo Tower in bright pink lights to raise awareness of breast health in a new and innovative way. The BCA campaign now illuminates more than 200 landmarks around the world each October. English actress, celebrity, and Estée Lauder spokesmodel Elizabeth Hurley has been working with Evelyn Lauder on breast cancer awareness since the mid-1990s and together they travel the world to raise awareness of the importance of breast health and early detection. In 1993, Evelyn Lauder founded the Breast Cancer Research Foundation (BCRF) as an independent, not-for-profit organization dedicated to funding innovative clinical and translational research. The BCRF has raised hundreds of millions of dollars and supports scientists across the USA, Canada, Latin America, Europe, the Middle East, and Australia. In partnership with Delta Airlines during National Breast Cancer Awareness Month, pink lemonade is served by flight attendants in pink dresses in a pink and white Boeing 757 decorated with the signature pink breast cancer ribbon. That's spreading the word.

STAND UP TO CANCER

When celebrities in television, film, sports, and music come together for the purpose of launching a one-hour telethon for cancer research you have a show that is guaranteed to make an impact. The show was hosted by three major USA TV networks and shown in 170 countries around the world on September 5, 2008. The charitable organization called Stand Up to Cancer (www.su2c.org), cofounded by nine dynamic women, received over $100 million in donations, 100% of which would go to facilitating what is commonly called bench to bedside research, or translational research. That is, the money would help move a newly developed compound or technology from research to the clinic by collaborative research teams.

One project that was funded by these donations is being led by Daniel Haber, doctor, researcher, and director of the Massachusetts General Hospital Cancer Center. Haber's team received $15 million to further develop a technology that allows the capture of metastasizing cancer cells, called circulating tumor cells (CTCs). The technology, called the CTC Chip, promises to reveal the crucial characteristics of CTCs that may provide a handle on how to stop metastasis. This is an exciting and novel area of research because previously researchers and doctors have concentrated on the primary tumor and not on the cells that migrate and spread; note that it is metastasis that causes 90% of cancer deaths. Because CTCs are captured from blood, the technology provides easy access to tumor cells; techniques that allow CTCs to be isolated may become the 'liquid biopsies' of tomorrow and replace the intrusive and often painful biopsies of today. The potential impact of such an easy procedure for diagnosis and treatment monitoring is huge. People are more likely to participate in cancer screening programs if they only need to give a sample of blood. More importantly, the time needed to see if a drug is working on a specific patient may be shortened because changes in CTC levels may be quicker and less expensive to observe compared to the shrinkage of a tumor. An earlier CTC detector called CellSearch has received US Food and Drug Administration (FDA) approval after clinical trials for the management of metastatic breast, colon, and prostate cancers but improvements to this earlier technology are in demand.

Stand Up to Cancer held a second broadcast on September 10, 2010 and raised an additional $80 million for cancer research.

SUSAN G. KOMEN FOR THE CURE

The power of love can spur one individual to achieve remarkable goals. This is evident in the story of the creation of the Susan G. Komen for the Cure organization. In a promise to her dying sister, Nancy G. Brinker said she would do everything in her power to end breast cancer. In 1982 she founded Susan G. Komen for the Cure, a global network of breast cancer survivors and activists dedicated to fighting breast cancer. They are now one of the largest non-government funders of breast cancer research in the world. They have also played a big part in public education. Being aware creates a club or team essence that allows members to talk, support, and do something for the cause. In addition to funding research for better treatments, Komen research grants also include research on why some tumors become resistant to drugs. Dr C. Kent Osborne, of the Baylor College of Medicine in Texas, has been a recipient of several Komen grants to investigate how tumors become resistant to tamoxifen, the gold-standard treatment for breast cancer.

MEDIKIDZ

Children with cancer have often been left out of the adult talk about cancer...until the small company called Medikidz was created. Medikidz offers education about many diseases, including cancer, using trendy modes of media. Superheroes, such as Pump, who knows about the heart, are used to explain medical concepts in comic-book formats. One such comic book, called *What's up with Bridget's Mum?*, explains breast cancer. The website www.medikidz.com provides a social networking site, online games, a virtual 3D body, and personal avatars. It also hosts calendars for treatment schedules. Business ideas that utilize internet technology are helping to break down the barriers of isolation.

WEB SERVICES

The web is providing opportunities for cancer patients to learn about their disease like never before. Although there may be too much information on invalid sites, patient information provided by national cancer institutes and societies is extensive. There are several services offered on the web that could only be dreamed about in the 1960s. The American Well Online Care service allows consumers to request a live online meeting with a physician who is able to review the patient's clinical information and prescribe medications. Of course, there are endless chat rooms and personal blogs to share personal experiences. The web will continue to play an important role in the cancer patient community for both medical information and moral support.

The era of Facebook, in which social networking is widespread, is beginning to contribute to the process of drug discovery. This fairly new type of communication has the potential to increase the global exchange of ideas, tools, and solutions. It allows individuals to contact groups or organizations that are working on similar problems. One site developed by Eli Lilly and Company, called Innocentive, encouraged the posting of specific technical problems within drug discovery and requested solutions from experts who had access to the site.

In addition, the use of video conferencing has facilitated 'webinars': seminars that you can view and participate in over the web. Such technology has also had an impact on training, including demonstrations of specialist surgical procedures.

RACES AND BIKE TOURS TO RAISE MONEY AND AWARENESS

Sports events, such as walks, runs, and bike tours, are common activities organized by charities to raise money and awareness. Race for Life, sponsored by Cancer Research UK, is one of the biggest charity fundraising events in the UK. Race for the Cure, sponsored by the Susan G. Komen Breast Cancer Foundation, began over 25 years ago in Dallas, Texas, with 800 runners. It now hosts over a million people a year in over 100 locations. The practice is spreading. Dr Michael Caligiuri, Director of the Ohio State University Comprehensive Cancer Center and Chief Executive Officer of the James Cancer Hospital, began exploring ways to fill gaps in funding for cancer research at the center. Instead of budget cuts, Dr Caligiuri decided that they would organize a bike event that would rely on the enthusiasm of sponsors and the community. In 2009, in a two-day event called Pelotonia, 2,265 people raised $4.5 million, all of which went to fund cancer research at the institution. And if anyone wants to know where Dr Caligiuri was during the event, he was, of course, on his bike covering the 180 miles, or 290 km, that he pledged to ride. The event was the first in a series of fundraising events. Raising funds independently gives money and power directly to cancer research.

CANCER SURVIVOR PARKS

Cancer survivors now hold an acheivement status. In their honor, the R.A. Bloch Cancer Foundation conceived and developed at least 20 cancer survivor parks across the USA and Canada. Their key message is: death and cancer are not synonymous. Each park contains three common elements in addition to unique features. The first element is a specific sculpture created by Victor Salmones that expresses the maze-like journey that cancer patients travel from diagnosis to recovery. The second is a 'Positive Attitude Walk' where visitors stroll and read plaques with suggestions on fighting cancer. The third element contains common sense advice to use during treatment. Having visited the Cancer Survivor Park in San Diego, California (Figure 18), I can confirm that the park radiates a unique positive serenity. You may not be surprised to hear that Richard Bloch was himself a survivor of a battle with lung cancer and vowed to help others with cancer for the rest of his life.

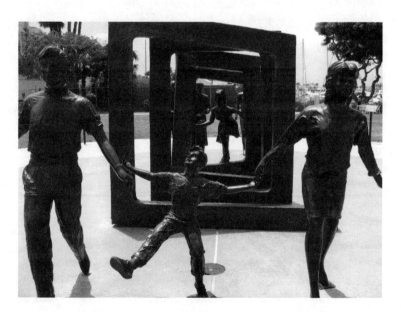

FIG 18 A Cancer Survivor Park, San Diego, California.

THE GOOD NEWS

The good news is that information about cancer is more easily accessible for all via telephone services and the web. People have formed organizations to raise awareness and funds for research. These have been powerful aids to progress in the field. Cancer scientists from around the globe have important forums that enable them to come together to discuss research strategies, build collaborations, and report results. Most importantly, cancer survivors are recognized and supported in the community.

11

HOW TO STARVE A TUMOR

...as a surgeon I had seen tumors and handled them, and saw that the blood vessels converging on the tumor by the thousands, and coming from a long distance, appeared to be new.

Judah Folkman, American medical scientist (1933–2008)

Julius Caesar, a general of the late Roman Republic, is remembered for his military brilliance. He often used siege warfare to mercilessly surround the city walls of his enemies to cut off food and supplies, and in this way starved whole cities. The strategy was also famously illustrated in the World War II battle at Stalingrad. Can research scientists borrow this strategy from military history and use it against cancer? That is, can they develop a treatment to cut off supplies (nutrients and oxygen) and starve a tumor?

What are the supply needs of cancer cells? A tumor is a quickly growing mass of cells that requires nutrients and oxygen supplied by the flow of blood through blood vessels. Cells can receive oxygen from a blood vessel by diffusion as long as they are less than 150 micrometers (that's 0.15 millimeters) from the vessel. Cells further away will be in an environment that has a lower-than-normal (or hypoxic) oxygen concentration. As a tumor grows, cells in the center of the tumor may become hypoxic and the need for supplies may increase. Tumors that spread to other parts of the body also need supplies. Recall that the ability of tumor cells to spread or metastasize is a defining characteristic of cancer. Metastasis is an unusual cell fate compared to the fate of most cells, as cells generally stay in one place. For example, lung cells stay in the lung and liver cells stay in the liver. Of course, there are a few exceptions such as blood cells and immune cells that travel throughout the body. The last step for a metastasizing cell is to set up a new colony or secondary tumor. The new colony needs to establish its own blood supply to receive oxygen and nutrients. Like a river being the lifeline of an early colony of America, the formation of new blood vessels is a tumor's lifeline in both hypoxic conditions and during metastasis.

One of the most important aspects that we have learned about a tumor is that it is not just a quiescent mass of rapidly dividing cells. Rather it has important and sometimes controlling interactions over its environment. Metastasized cells can actually convert the cells of a local blood vessel to grow towards the newly colonizing tumor. The new growth of blood vessel cells forms a branch from the existing vessel, similar to the growth of a branch from a tree trunk. This process of the formation of new blood vessels from pre-existing blood vessels is called **angiogenesis.**

A visionary strategy for cancer therapies was postulated in 1971 by one of the fathers of the study of angiogenesis, Judah Folkman (Folkman, 1971). Folkman, an American surgeon and researcher, hypothesized that if we could shut off a tumor's blood supply and starve a tumor we would cause the death of tumor cells. In other words, blocking angiogenesis is a strategy for developing cancer therapies. Angiogenesis, though important during embryonic development, is mostly absent in the healthy adult. The fact that angiogenesis is important for a tumor but is not crucial in the healthy adult makes it attractive as a therapeutic target since blocking the process is expected to have few side-effects. Another advantage of blocking angiogenesis as an anti-cancer strategy is that the drug will be targeting normal blood vessel cells and not genetically unstable and mutating cancer cells, so the development of drug resistance should be minimal.

THE ANGIOGENIC SWITCH

Basic science underpins clinical applications. To begin working towards the development of anti-angiogenic drugs, we had to learn how the process of angiogenesis occurs and how it is normally restricted in the healthy adult. Around this time, Folkman and others formulated the concept of the angiogenic switch. The angiogenic switch described a system in which there are molecules produced by cells that work to block angiogenesis and other molecules produced by cells that work to promote angiogenesis. If the activity of the angiogenic blockers is more than that of the promoters, then angiogenesis is inhibited. When the activity of the promoters outweighs that of the blockers then angiogenesis occurs. It is the balance of the activity of the two opposing families of molecules that decides whether the process of angiogenesis is on or off. Under most conditions in the adult, the switch is off. In cancer, tumors produce promoting factors and this tips the balance of the

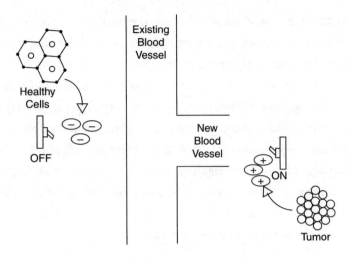

FIG 19 The angiogenic switch.

angiogenic switch towards the 'on' mode, triggering the sprouting of new blood vessels from existing blood vessels (see Figure 19).

So how could the formation of new blood vessels be blocked, shutting off a tumor's blood supply? The angiogenic switch provides us with two types of molecules to work with when thinking of strategies for drug design: promoters and blockers. One way is to block the promoting signals produced by the tumor and prevent them from signaling to the pre-existing vessels. The molecular signals needed to be identified and the mechanisms of how they work needed to be understood. All the tools and techniques needed to isolate and clone these factors were at hand for researchers at this time. One major player that promotes angiogenesis, called vascular endothelial growth factor (VEGF), was identified. Although other growth factors were shown to promote angiogenesis, VEGF is specific to endothelial (blood vessel) cells. VEGF binds to a VEGF receptor on the endothelial cell surface and triggers a signaling pathway that is very similar to the epithelial growth factor (EGF) growth factor receptor described in detail in Chapter 4. The receptor belongs to the tyrosine kinase receptor family and many of the molecules used to pass the signal to the nucleus are the same as in the EGF signaling pathway (e.g. RAS, MAPK). Ultimately, VEGF induces the growth of endothelial cells. Proteins that block angiogenesis, such as endostatin and angiostatin, were also identified.

HEROES

One hero of the field of angiogenesis is Judah Folkman, mentioned above as one of fathers of the study of angiogenesis. In addition to his early hypothesis regarding the potential to treat cancer by blocking angiogenesis, the late Judah Folkman made many other contributions to this entirely new field of basic and clinical research which he founded. As examples, he created experimental systems that allowed the investigation of the sequential steps involved in blood vessel formation, and also contributed to the use of thalidomide and other anti-angiogenic cancer therapies, as discussed below. Folkman was elected to the National Academy of Sciences in 1990.

Another hero in this story is Napoleone Ferrara, an Italian physician who has been employed by the pharmaceutical giant Genentech since 1988. It was here that he isolated and studied VEGF. One of the tools that Ferrara was using to study this molecule was an antibody against VEGF. Antibodies are made in the body as part of an immune response to a foreign invader, such as bacteria. Specific antibodies for research can be made by mice after exposing the animal to a specific antigen. In this case, human VEGF was injected into mice. After several weeks immune cells that produce specific antibodies to VEGF are isolated and modified so they can be grown in a laboratory *in vitro* (meaning 'in glass', or in a test tube, outside of the body) and the desired antibodies can be harvested. Antibodies can be tagged with fluorescent markers to become visible and used to track and locate the molecules that they bind. They can also be used to block a molecule's activity to study its function. To Ferrara and his colleagues' surprise, the mouse antibody to VEGF inhibited tumor growth in animal models. Not only was this exciting from a therapeutic perspective, because it showed for the first time that tumor growth was dependent on angiogenesis, but it also identified VEGF as a major player in angiogenesis. VEGF is *the* 'blood vessel maker'. Researchers now had a target (VEGF and its signaling pathway) to aim for in order to develop a new drug designed to block angiogenesis and starve a tumor.

THE DEVELOPMENT OF ANTI-ANGIOGENIC DRUGS

The early experiments conducted by Ferrara and colleagues paved the way to the development of Avastin (generic name bevacizumab; made by Genentech), the first anti-angiogenic drug to be approved to treat cancer. Antibodies are extremely specific for their target antigens and are attractive therapeutic agents that can easily reach specific molecules outside of the cell. The strategy used by Ferrara and his colleagues was to design a specific antibody to VEGF that would be similar to the research tool that he used in his mouse studies and that could be used as a drug in humans.

A mouse antibody would cause an immune response in humans and so could not be used as a drug. By using molecular techniques, a humanized antibody, Avastin, was made by grafting the main part of a human antibody to regions of the mouse antibody that specifically recognized human VEGF. Humanization of an antibody overcomes immune rejection of a 'foreign' mouse antibody when used in humans. Avastin works by binding to VEGF and preventing the binding of VEGF to its receptor. This approach stops angiogenesis at a first major step. After demonstrating success in clinical trials in combination with chemotherapy, the drug Avastin was approved by the US Food and Drug Administration (FDA) and the European Commission for the treatment of colorectal cancer, and later for treatment of advanced breast, kidney, and lung cancers. Its use is currently restricted in the UK where a threshold is set for cost-effectiveness of new cancer therapies.

Several other approaches that aimed to target angiogenic promoters were developed. The new breast cancer drugs targeted at the EGF receptor taught us that receptors for growth factors are 'druggable' targets: that is, they are molecules that can be blocked by a drug to give a clinical response. Most growth factor receptors are kinase receptors and their kinase activity can be blocked by selective small molecule inhibitors. In the case of the VEGF receptor, such kinase inhibitors will prevent the receptor from passing the VEGF signal into the cell and will inhibit the growth of endothelial cells and ultimately angiogenesis. Two multi-kinase inhibitors that target the VEGF receptor, Nexavar (generic name sorafenib; manufactured by Bayer Pharm) and Sutent (sunitinib; made by Pfizer), have been approved for the treatment of kidney cancer. In summary, Avastin and the drugs mentioned above

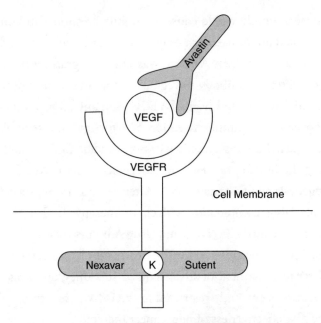

FIG 20 Anti-angiogenic drugs that target VEGF and its receptor. Drugs are shaded; 'K' represents the Kinase domain of VEGFR.

target and block the angiogenic promoter VEGF and its receptor (Figure 20).

Another strategy for developing anti-angiogenic drugs is to administer blockers of angiogenesis. Endostatin is an inhibitor that is found naturally in the body. The administration of endostatin manufactured in the laboratory became another therapeutic candidate and was the first inhibitor to be tested in clinical trials. Unfortunately, endostatin did not show a clinical benefit in clinical trials and the development of the drug was discontinued in the USA. Endostatin was approved in China in 2005. There is a possibility that the failure of the drug to exhibit a response in US clinical trials was due to the design of the trial rather than it being truly ineffective. The drug showed a positive effect in animals for early-stage cancer but in the clinical trials the drug was tested on patients with advanced cancer. In other words, if the drug is most effective for early-stage cancer, its result would not be seen in a trial that uses patients with advanced cancer. Other natural and synthetic inhibitors of angiogenesis are being developed as cancer drugs and several are in early clinical trials.

A BAD DRUG TURNED GOOD

Many people have heard the horrific story of thalidomide. Thalidomide was a drug, first marketed in Germany in 1956, which was prescribed to women for morning sickness. The horror was that the drug was a **teratogen** (an agent that causes birth defects) and caused severe birth abnormalities, including characteristic limb deformities, in the children of mothers who took the drug during pregnancy. Over 10,000 children worldwide were born with thalidomide-induced developmental defects. Evidence suggests that it is thalidomide's anti-angiogenic properties that are responsible for the limb defects of children born to mothers treated with thalidomide. In 2006, thalidomide was approved for the first time by the FDA as part of a combination therapy for a cancer of the bone marrow called multiple myeloma. Analogs of thalidomide with reduced toxicity have been developed. One of these new derivatives, Revlimid (generic name lenalidamide), has also received FDA approval for the treatment of multiple myeloma. The teratogenic effects of these drugs will not be a concern to many cancer patients because cancer usually strikes after one's child-bearing years. Otherwise, patient education regarding pregnancy is crucial. Although the mechanisms by which thalidomide and its derivatives exert their therapeutic effects are still largely unknown, their anti-angiogenic activity may be a contributing factor.

HYPOXIA PROMOTES ANGIOGENESIS

The body has remarkable mechanisms with which to protect itself. In conditions of low concentrations of oxygen (hypoxia), angiogenesis is triggered. Many contact-lens wearers may have experienced the induction of angiogenesis due to hypoxia first hand, as I did. In the early days of contact lenses it was acceptable to go to sleep wearing your contact lenses. At a routine visit to the optometrist, I was told that I had blood vessels growing in my eye and was interrogated about when and how often I wore the contact lenses. He patiently explained that when you sleep your closed eyelid combined with the additional barrier of the contact lens cause a reduction in oxygen available to the eye. Instead of eye cells dying because of the lack of oxygen, the growth of new blood vessels was induced to meet the increased need for oxygen. I no longer wear my contact lenses when I go to sleep.

The tumor environment is often the site of hypoxia, and, similar to the above scenario, stimulates angiogenesis. The biochemistry behind this response is fascinating because an enzyme acts as a direct oxygen sensor. The enzyme 'accessorizes' the main player in this story, a transcription factor called hypoxia-inducible factor (or HIF) that turns on genes whose products are important for angiogenesis. One can probably now guess that one of the genes turned on by transcription factor HIF is the *VEGF* gene. Under normal concentrations of oxygen a specific enzyme, called prolyl-4-hydroxylase, adds an hydroxyl group (OH) to HIF. This accessory ultimately tags HIF for destruction so that it is not available to turn on genes such as the *VEGF* gene. Thus, under normal oxygen concentrations angiogenesis is inhibited. Under hypoxia, however, the specific enzyme is unable to add an hydroxyl group to HIF and therefore it is not tagged for destruction. Transcription factor HIF is available to turn on its target genes, including the *VEGF* gene, and angiogenesis is triggered. This pathway will likely be targeted by future cancer therapies to inhibit angiogenesis.

THE GOOD NEWS

The good news is that there are now several anti-angiogenic drugs, in addition to Avastin, that have been approved as cancer therapeutics, and over 80 such drugs are in clinical trials. The arsenal of weapons against cancer is growing. Mark McClellan, the Commissioner of the FDA, announced in 2004 that 'antiangiogenic therapy can now be considered the fourth modality of cancer treatment' in addition to surgery, radiotherapy, and chemotherapy. In general, anti-angiogenic drugs are well tolerated. Note that the effects of many of the approved anti-angiogenic drugs on extending progression-free survival and/or overall survival of the patient are modest and measurable in months rather than years. Some patients respond better than others to Avastin, suggesting that tumor genotype may play a role in how a patient will respond to the drug. Also, the positive effects of Avastin have been demonstrated in combination with chemotherapies. There is still a lot to learn about tumor angiogenesis. We hopefully await improved benefits from anti-angiogenic drug candidates now in clinical trials and from new therapeutic combinations.

The fruits of studying angiogenesis extend beyond cancer and have laid the foundation for the development of drugs for other diseases such as ocular disease. The FDA-approved anti-VEGF antibody, Lucentis, accounts for 40% of patients who are blind from age-related macular degeneration regaining their sight within months of treatment.

12

A VACCINE AGAINST CERVICAL CANCER

> Discovering that a virus is the central cause of a cancer provides
> an exceptional opportunity to prevent that cancer by preventing
> the initiating virus infection. It certainly is good news that a simple
> series of vaccinations now available will likely reduce a young
> woman's risk of developing the second most frequent cause of
> cancer deaths in women by at least 70%.
>
> *John Schiller, PhD, Senior Investigator, National Cancer Institute,*
> *National Institutes of Health*

Medicines, when they are fully effective and without side-effects, can be astonishing, but wouldn't medical approaches for the prevention of cancer be the ultimate solution? It may sound like fantasy but let's look at a chapter from the history of medicine. Diseases that were once dreaded in the past are now kept at bay with vaccines. We are familiar with vaccines against smallpox, mumps, measles, and polio. The story of the development of the smallpox vaccine is remarkable. Smallpox is caused by the variola virus and is an extremely contagious disease. Symptoms include a severe rash that produces scarring, and a high fever. The term 'small pockes' was first used in England in the late 1400s to distinguish it from 'great pockes', the disease now called syphilis. Smallpox proved fatal for approximately 30% of those who contracted the disease and has killed millions of people over the centuries. There is no treatment. The outlook was grim, but in 1796 the scene was set to change.

In early attempts to protect people from smallpox, **variolation** or inoculation was practiced. The procedure involved taking material from lesions of smallpox patients and introducing it subcutaneously on the arms or legs of a non-immune person. This procedure usually provided immunity during exposure to smallpox later in life. Variolation laid the foundation for the significant breakthrough made by Edward Jenner, an English physician, who translated an observation into a new medical practice. The observation was that milkmaids who had been infected with cowpox from cows did not develop smallpox. Cowpox is a skin disease commonly transmitted from the udders of infected cows to the hands of milkmaids; cowpox is caused by a virus related to the variola virus that causes smallpox. In a new medical procedure, Jenner inoculated a small boy with cowpox to induce immunity against smallpox. The new medical procedure gave birth to vaccination. The success of compulsory and targeted smallpox vaccination programs in future generations led to the announcement by the World Health Organization in 1980 that smallpox had been eradicated. Variations of Jenner's procedure gave birth to great medical advances that now prevent many different diseases and saved billions of lives over the following centuries. Recently we have added specific cancers to the list of diseases that vaccines can prevent. The first vaccines against cervical cancer are the focus of this chapter.

As mentioned in Chapter 8, the worldwide cervical cancer burden is heavy, accounting for 300,000 deaths per year. Over 200,000 of these deaths occur in the developing world, with particularly high rates in Eastern Africa and South Africa (Plate 5). It is in these regions where screening is not easily available that a vaccine may be most effective in reducing the number of deaths by cervical cancer.

WHY DOES A VACCINE WORK AGAINST CERVICAL CANCER?

One may ask, 'why does a vaccine work against cervical cancer?' The answer is simple. Because 100% of cervical cancers are caused by a virus called human papillomavirus (HPV). And so we can approach the prevention of cervical cancer like many diseases caused by a viral agent: by vaccination. Note that 80% of all cancers are not caused by an infectious agent as far as we know, and so for this larger subset of cancers a preventative vaccine is not yet an option.

HPV is the most common type of sexually transmitted viral infection. More than 50% of men and women who are sexually active acquire HPV infection during their lifetime. Note that not all HPV infections lead to cancer. Usually, the infection is cleared by your immune system. But when an HPV infection is *not* cleared, it becomes a long-term (chronic) infection. Chronic HPV infection is the central risk factor for cervical cancer. The time between acquiring the infection and developing cancer can be 10 years or more. Note that of the 130 different types of HPV, only a small number is considered 'high risk' for cervical cancer. In fact, only two types, HPV16 and HPV18, account for 70% of all cervical cancers. One out of 10 women infected with high-risk HPV will develop a chronic infection that may lead to cervical cancer.

The virus infects dividing cells in the deeper layers of the lining of the cervix through tiny tears and abrasions. Over time the viral DNA becomes part of the cell's DNA and uses the cell machinery to produce viral oncogenic proteins. These proteins bind to and degrade important tumor suppressor proteins, such as P53 and retinoblastoma (RB) (discussed in Chapter 3) and the development of cancer is triggered.

HOW DOES THE VACCINE WORK?

The basis of many preventative vaccines is to introduce an inactive or genetically weakened (attenuated) form of the disease-causing agent into a person to trigger an immune response. In the case of the vaccines developed against HPV, the major structural protein that forms the 'framework' of the virus, called L1, is the key. The viral L1 gene can be expressed in cells. The protein product self-assembles into virus-like particles and is used as the basis of the vaccine. This strategy is safe because these virus-like particles do not contain the viral genome, which include the viral oncogenes that are involved in cancer development. Virus-like particles are not able to replicate. A viral-like particle is similar to an empty crab shell; the external appearance is the same as if there was a crab inside but there is no life within it. The self-assembly aspect of

L1 is important because it provides a structure that is similar to the authentic virus and provides a design for the immune system to target. The idea is to generate antibodies against the outer surface of the virus-like particle that in the future can bind to the outer surface of an incoming virus and thereby prevent it from infecting its target cell. In addition to the inactive form of the disease-causing agent, some vaccines include an additive to enhance the immune response, called an **adjuvant**.

Two HPV vaccines have been developed commercially: Gardasil (Merck) and Cervarix (GlaxoSmithKline). Gardasil was the world's first cervical cancer vaccine, approved in June 2006 by the US Food and Drug Administration (FDA). Gardasil prevents cervical cancer caused by HPV16 and HPV18, as well as genital warts caused by HPV6 and HPV11. Remember, HPV16 and HPV18 account for 70% of all cervical cancers. HPV6 and HPV11 cause 90% of genital warts cases. Note that genital warts can be similar to precancerous changes and may lead to false-positive results during screening. So Gardasil targets real villains of cervical cancer, HPV16 and HPV18, and also two imposters, HPV6 and HPV11, and it prevents two distinct diseases of HPV infection, cervical cancer and genital warts. Cervarix was designed to specifically prevent cervical cancer caused by HPV16 and HPV18. It has been approved in many countries including members of the European Union and Australia and has been chosen for use in the UK national vaccination program. It was approved in the USA in 2009. The two vaccines use L1 virus-like particles as described above but they have different adjuvants (the immune-boosting ingredients). Gardasil uses alum (aluminum salts) and Cervarix uses a proprietary adjuvant called AS04. AS04 contains alum and a new component, monophospholipid A

(MPL). MPL is derived from an extract of Gram-negative bacterial cell walls and stimulates the immune system in ways that simple aluminum salts do not. It has been suggested that uncertainty about the new adjuvant is one of the reasons that the FDA delayed its decision regarding approval of Cervarix for over 2 years.

WHO SHOULD RECEIVE THE VACCINE?

It is important to stress that the vaccines discussed in this chapter are preventative vaccines and are only effective *before* HPV infection. They are not therapeutic vaccines that act to treat an infection, and so it is important to vaccinate before people are exposed to the virus; that is, before they become sexually active. Objections have arisen from some families because any implication of children being sexually active is not welcome. It is not essential that a 13-year-old girl understands the details of *why* she needs the vaccine to prevent cervical cancer before she receives it. That is, young girls really do not need to understand that an infection transmitted by sexual contact could cause cervical cancer many years later; they will grow into this knowledge. The important thing is that a young girl accepts to have the vaccine under her parents' guidance and understands that it is beneficial to her health. Perhaps with time and education, people will show less resistance towards their children receiving the vaccine, knowing that it will be guarding against a cancer that is not always easy to detect and can be painful to treat.

In the UK, the HPV vaccination program began in September 2008 and offered the Cervarix vaccine to all 12–13- and 17–18-year-old girls. Afterwards, a 'catch-up' program extended the offer to vaccinate girls between 13 and 18 years of age. Parental consent is required. Vaccination involves receiving three injections over six months. Studies demonstrate that the vaccine is preventative for at least six years but ongoing research will address the period of time that the vaccine remains effective. The US Centers for Disease Control and Prevention (CDC) recommends that all girls aged 11 or 12 years should be given either the Cervarix or Gardasil vaccine. They also recommend catch-up vaccination for girls and young women from 13 to 26 years if they have not already received the recommended three doses. There is not enough evidence of benefit at the present time for recommending vaccination of all women who are older than 26. Although the CDC has not added either vaccine to the recommended list of routine vaccines for boys, Gardasil has been approved for the prevention of genital warts in boys. Boys and young men aged 9–26 years are at liberty to choose to get the vaccine to prevent genital warts.

Unfortunately, there are some forms of media that feed on sensationalism and this has been a destructive force in public health with regards to vaccinations. The misinformed reports of a link between the measles, mumps, and rubella (MMR) vaccine and autism has resulted in the rise of diseases we should not need to be concerned with in the 21st century. The first attack on the cervical cancer vaccine has already occurred. It was a front-page headline reporting the death of a teenage girl shortly after receiving the cervical cancer vaccine. The next day, in a much smaller article printed beyond the front page, it was reported that the teenager's death was due to an underlying condition and not the cervical cancer vaccine. However, the initial report did some damage and caused some panic. It is important for readers to question attention-grabbing media coverage of medical issues. In this case it is worth bearing in mind how many doses of the cervical cancer vaccine have already been given without incident.

HEROES

Although there are hundreds of contributors to the development of the cervical cancer vaccines, there are three exceptional heroes behind the science of such vaccines who are worthy of mention. Harald zur Hausen, a German scientist, received global recognition with the award of the Nobel Prize in Physiology or Medicine in 2008 for proving that HPVs cause cervical cancer. Although zur Hausen presented some data in 1974 suggesting that HPV was the cause of cervical cancer, it was to take another decade and the use of molecular approaches to accumulate enough evidence for it to be accepted. The existence of several HPV types, some playing a role in cervical cancer and other types not, clouded the investigation. It was the isolation and detection of HPV16 and HPV18 in 70% of cervical cancer biopsies that made the evidence irrefutable.

Two other heroes, Douglas Lowy and John Schiller from the USA, showed that the L1 protein of the virus could assemble into virus-like particles that could elicit antibodies that prevented virus infection of cells grown in the laboratory, and took their finding into Phase I clinical trials. Lowry and Schiller also did an experiment similar to that performed by Jenner many years ago, but with animal models. Initially there was a problem because HPV would not infect other animal species. So they used cottontail rabbit papillomavirus in domestic rabbits and bovine papillomavirus in cows. When they injected species-specific viral-like particles into animals they observed that these animals were protected from later experimental exposure to the same species-specific virus. The success of these studies paved the way to testing the approach in humans in clinical trials. Lowy and Schiller were presented with the Landon Award at the 100th anniversary of the American Association for Cancer Research in 2007.

THE GOOD NEWS

The good news is that the HPV vaccine will prevent 70% of cervical cancers in vaccinated populations. Since it takes a decade or two between HPV infection and the development of cervical cancer we will not be able to observe the full benefits of vaccination until this length of time has passed. One may question whether vaccination is needed in the developed world, where cervical cancer has been controlled by Pap screening. One answer is that the prevention of HPV infection by the vaccine will abolish the need for the sometimes painful treatment or removal of precancerous cells and early cancers. As mentioned in Chapter 9, Pap screening will still be necessary to prevent the 30% of cervical cancers that are not protected against by the current cervical cancer vaccines. This point needs to be emphasized: women must continue with Pap screening. Studies have shown that a proportion of women carry multiple infections from different types of HPV. Because of the relative ease of implementation, the vaccine has the potential of having even greater benefit in low-resource settings where Pap screening and appropriate after-treatment are not available.

THE FUTURE OF PREVENTATIVE
CANCER VACCINES

The rates of certain types of oral cancer among men and women are rising at an alarming rate in Europe, the USA, and other developed countries. This was surprising because use of tobacco and alcohol, previous known causes of oral cancers, is declining. The missing piece of the puzzle is that HPV infection, transmitted by oral sex, has been shown to be the cause of a subset of head and neck cancers. It is fortuitous that HPV16, which is causative for cervical cancer, is also causative for oral cancers. HPV16 is found in 84% of HPV-positive oral cancers. Thus, the vaccines that have been developed to prevent cervical cancer may have a wider application than originally thought. Head and neck cancers affect men and women. This fact also brings support to the suggestion that men should also be vaccinated against HPV infection.

Cervical cancer vaccines were not the first vaccines targeted to prevent a specific cancer. Hepatitis B vaccine was the first vaccine against a cancer and the first against a sexually transmitted infection. A national vaccination program against Hepatitis B virus was initiated in Taiwan as early as 1984 to prevent cirrhosis and liver cancer. Like cervical cancer, development of liver cancer is dependent upon chronic viral infection. Before the vaccination program was initiated 16% of all cancer deaths were due to liver cancer caused by Hepatitis B. The program has been a success and studies have demonstrated that a majority of liver cancers in children can be prevented by vaccination. This result is sensational and prompted the World Health Organization to recommend global Hepatitis B vaccination programs. The USA, Canada, South Africa, and many countries in Western Europe have put Hepatitis B vaccination programs in place and have reported significant impact. A robust safety record is demonstrated since 1982, after more than a billion doses of vaccine have been given. Continued and expanded implementation of these programs could lead to the elimination of Hepatitis B.

Tumors can appear very different from host cells because of an accumulation of mutations and the appearance of tumor-specific proteins on their surface (tumor-specific antigens). With a stretch of imagination, they may even be viewed to be similar to foreign infectious agents. Creating vaccines that target not an infectious agent but instead tumor-specific surface proteins is an area that is undergoing active research and which has shown some success in preclinical trials. It is hoped that one day we may be able to stimulate the body's own immune response to guard against tumor cells in the same way that it can be stimulated to guard against infective agents.

13

A FIT LIKE A GLOVE

We've made considerable progress towards our goal of better, safer treatments. Now we need to take the next big step, by matching targeted treatments to the altered genes in each patient's cancer.

Harpal Kumar, Chief Executive Officer, Cancer Research UK

Progress is moving us towards 'personalized medicine'. What does it really mean? These days we can personalize many things: wardrobes, car license plates, tattoos, and screen savers. But the most personalized item a person can possess is their individual genome. No two people are exactly the same genetically (except identical twins). Only cancer patients have a more personalized item, and that is the genome of their tumors. The DNA of tumors has evolved compared to the genome present in the rest of the individual. Tumor DNA has recorded the evidence of damage by carcinogens in the form of mutations. The mutations confer cell advantages for survival in the same way as described by Darwin's theory of evolution. In some cases, it is this variability among tumor genes that determines whether a cancer drug works on some people but not on others. For decades, most treatment options have been based on physical attributes of the tumor, mainly size and location, without taking into account the vastly different genetic make-up of tumors. It is not surprising then that one treatment may work for some patients and not for others. The concept is similar to that of fitting clothes. The more information a tailor possesses about his client (waist size, hip size, leg length, etc.), the more likely the garment will fit like a glove. 'One size fits all' rarely works for all. Personalized medicine is medicine tailored for the individual. In simple terms, personalized medicine is about matching the right drug with the right patient at the right time. It promises to eliminate the hit-and-miss approach whereby a doctor tries a drug and, after it fails, he tries another, and then another, by which time the tumor has a stronghold. Personalized medicine also promises to select those who will benefit from a harsh regime of chemotherapy from those who will not. This information will guide doctors to administer chemotherapy only to those who will benefit, sparing those who will not benefit the toxic side-effects of the drug.

PERSONALIZED MEDICINE
FOR BREAST CANCER

Personalized medicine has been used to a limited extent for decades in the case of breast cancer. Upon diagnosis, a breast tumor is tested and classified as estrogen-receptor-positive or -negative. Estrogen is a sex hormone that acts as a growth factor via estrogen receptors in breast cells. The growth of estrogen-receptor-positive (ER+) cells can be blocked by drugs that interfere with the estrogen/estrogen-receptor pathway. Breast cancers that are not ER+ will not respond to these types of drugs.

Two strategies are currently used to target ER+ breast cancers. One strategy is to block the binding of estrogen to its receptor. Tamoxifen, a drug in use for more than 30 years, competes with estrogen for receptor binding. When tamoxifen binds to the estrogen receptor it prevents estrogen binding and estrogen-receptor signaling and thus blocks breast cancer growth.

The second strategy involves blocking the body's production of estrogen in post-menopausal women by targeting an estrogen-synthesizing enzyme, which is called aromatase. Note that this strategy is only appropriate in post-menopausal women, in whom aromatase in fat cells is the main source of estrogen. It is not appropriate in premenopausal women, in whom estrogen is produced mainly by the ovaries. Aromatase inhibitors, including exemestane, anastrozole, and letrozole, are effective for ER+ tumors. Use of both tamoxifen and aromatase inhibitors is called hormone therapy.

The evolution of personalized medicine for breast cancer has advanced beyond testing only for the estrogen receptor. Testing for the presence of too much HER2, a molecule related to epidermal growth factor (EGF) receptor, is another indicator for the best choice of treatment. Patients whose tumors have an abundance of HER2 are more likely to benefit from the drug Herceptin (generic name trastuzumab). Herceptin is a human-made antibody that works by binding to HER2 (discussed in Chapter 5).

Even more exciting breakthroughs are on the horizon. A strategy that uses molecular combinations is being developed to target breast cancer cells, not healthy cells, in patients with breast cancer susceptibility due to germline *BRCA1* and *BRCA2* gene mutations. These patients have inherited a mutation in one of the two copies of the *BRCA1/2* genes. Tumors in these patients develop when a second mutation occurs in a cell, blocking a specific DNA-repair pathway. These cells are viable because they use a back-up DNA-repair pathway. But when a drug called olaparib (an agent called a PARP inhibitor) that targets this pathway is given, cancer cells undergo cell death. Healthy cells contain only one *BRCA1/2* mutation and do not need a back-up DNA-repair pathway and so they should not be affected by a drug that blocks the back-up. This strategy, which uses molecular partners to create a deadly combination, is called synthetic lethality. Encouraging results from early-phase clinical trials have been reported in the *New England Journal of Medicine* (Fong et al., 2009).

The use of chemotherapy after surgery is commonly prescribed, yet not all women with early-stage breast cancer may benefit equally. There is a concern that some of these patients may have a low risk of the cancer returning and may be over-treated, enduring the harsh side-effects of chemotherapy without need.

Oncotype DX21 is a test that analyzes the expression of 21 genes demonstrated to be involved in breast cancer. Expression of both the *ER* and *HER2* genes are included in the test. The results of the test help to calculate the risk of the cancer returning (recurrence score) and predict the likelihood that a patient with early-stage breast cancer will respond to chemotherapy. The implications for patients with low (less than 17) or high (31 or higher) recurrence scores are clear, sparing those who will not benefit from chemotherapy and selecting those who are likely to benefit. The test is listed in the National Comprehensive Cancer Network *Breast Cancer*

Guidelines (2008) as an option to help guide chemotherapy treatment decisions and is being used around the world with sales in 55 countries. It is available in the UK in the private sector. The TAILORx Breast Cancer Trial (see National Cancer Institute, *Fact Sheet TAILORx*, in the Bibliography) will use this methodology on 10,000 women in the USA and Canada and evaluate the effects of chemotherapy for women with midrange recurrence scores. This trial the first of its kind, in that it is looking at treatment based on an individual's risk.

It is likely that similar tests will be developed for other cancers. The Oncotype DX Colon Cancer Test analyzes the expression of 12 genes and predicts the risk of colon cancer recurrence (but not treatment response). Part of the improvements observed for breast cancer treatment is due to molecular sub-classifications. That is, we can identify different types of breast cancer based on molecular characterization (e.g. ER+, HER+, etc.). Other cancers, such as prostate cancer, lack molecular sub-classifications and are more difficult to treat. As our understanding of tumor genes grows and as we continue to create drugs that target specific molecules based on our understanding, personalized medicine will become more efficient at matching the right drug to the right patient and will become applicable to more types of cancer.

TUMOR MUTATIONS CAN ENHANCE OR BLOCK DRUG RESPONSES

The advent of molecularly targeted drugs led us to understand that the desired drug target may be altered by mutation in some patients. That is, gene mutations underlying cancer development may lead to a change in the structure and/or function of the gene product (possibly the drug target). In Chapter 5 the growth factor receptor called EGF receptor was discussed as a target of a host of new drugs. You may remember that targeting the part of the receptor molecule on the outside of the cell with antibodies and the active site of the receptor located on the inside of the cell with small molecules are both successful strategies. One drug using the latter strategy, Iressa (generic name gefitinib), was developed (and approved in the USA and Japan) for the treatment of a subtype of lung cancer. During clinical trials Iressa only seemed to work in about 10% of cases. But when it worked, it worked very well and tumor regression was clear. The results were confusing and caused some researchers to want to abandon the drug's development. We have since learned that patients who respond to Iressa have tumors that carry a specific mutation in the EGF receptor gene, *EGFR*. The mutations cause the receptors to be hyperactive, and at the same time cause the tumor cells to be more vulnerable to Iressa.

In contrast, tumor DNA that carries a mutation in a gene called *KRAS* blocks the success of the drug Erbitux (generic name cetuximab). Erbitux is an antibody against EGF receptor that can be used to treat EGF-receptor-expressing metastatic colon cancer, except in patients who carry a *KRAS* mutation. Patients with a *KRAS* mutation will not respond to this drug. Recalling the details of the EGF pathway (illustrated in Chapter 5) helps to understand why patients with *KRAS* mutations will not respond. It comes down to the chain of command of carrying the signal: the EGF receptor is the first molecule to receive the EGF signal. If EGF receptor is the oncogenic signaling molecule of a cancer, then blocking it will be a successful strategy. But if a molecule further down the chain of command is the 'broken cog', or oncogenic signaling molecule, then blocking the EGF receptor will be in vain. It is like shooting the wrong messenger. *KRAS* is mutated and acts as the broken cog in about 40% of colorectal cancer patients. In 2009, the US Food and Drug Administration (FDA) updated the Erbitux label to include a recommendation on screening for the *KRAS* mutation. This is one of the first cases where **pharmacogenomic** information (meaning the influence of genetic variation on a drug's response) is included on a drug label. Recommendations for *KRAS* mutation testing is also included for a similar drug called Vectibix (panitumumab). Testing for *KRAS* mutations is a paradigm shift in deciding the best treatment for colorectal cancer. These examples illustrate the concept that knowing the genetic make-up of a tumor helps doctors to choose the best treatment for an individual.

BIOBANKS, PERSONAL BIOSAMPLES, AND CANCER RESEARCH

Cancer patients and the general population are now becoming part, literally, of the team in the fight against cancer. The last decade has seen the development of **biobanks**, large collections of human biological tissue and associated health information that will become an unprecedented resource for future research. *Time* magazine listed biobanks as one of the 'top 10 ideas changing the world right now' (Park, 2009). Similar to the call for donating blood to help others, participating in biobanks is crucial. This is because good-quality, properly prepared, and correctly stored human tissue is the limiting but ultimate research resource.

Biobanks can be disease-specific or general. The US National Cancer Institute cancer Human Biobank (caHUB) is a national project that will focus on cancer. Several smaller and independent general biobanks, such as the Mayo Clinic Biobank and Genetics Alliance Biobank, also exist in the USA. Iceland, Japan, Sweden, and the UK have national biobanks that are based on the general population. The participation in Iceland is notable in that 60% of the population have given samples to the deCODE Genetics project. Using an invitation system, the UK Biobank reached its initial target of recruiting 500,000 people aged 40–69 (UK Biobank, www. ukbiobank.ac.uk/). The participants were asked to give saliva, blood, and urine samples along with permission to access their medical records, held by the UK National Health Service. The National Health Service is well placed in that it treats the single largest group of people in the world and keeps health records on individuals from birth to death. Please consider giving 'a little piece of yourself' for future generations if you have an opportunity to participate in a biobank.

Organizers of clinical trials are beginning to ask patients for permission to collect fresh biopsies that will help scientists to catalog mutations that occur in specific cancers and to monitor which profiles respond to specific treatments. These patients are contributing to knowledge that will benefit future generations. Here's one example. In general, lung cancer patients are treated in a 'one-size-fits-all'-type manner. In a landmark clinical trial called BATTLE (which stands for Biomarker-integrated Approaches of Targeted Therapy for Lung Cancer Elimination), conducted at the M.D. Anderson Cancer Center, Houston, Texas, the effectiveness of a personalized medicine approach was tested to treat patients with lung cancer. This was made possible by the information obtained from fresh patient biopsies. The trial, led by Edward S. Kim, was unique because the knowledge gained early on in the trial, with regards to what genetic profiles did best with a particular drug, was used to assign patients to particular drugs later on. Overall, the conclusions supported the idea that targeted drugs are superior to chemotherapy for patients with specific activating mutations in targeted molecules.

SEQUENCING OF THE CANCER GENOME

We are lucky that it is becoming more feasible to be able to test genes of an individual's tumor with the great advances of technology that has occurred over the last two decades. The first human genome project cost $1.5 billion and took 15 years to complete. Since this Herculean effort technology has advanced and in 2007 allowed the first complete genomic sequencing of one individual. The project was completed within two months and for under a million dollars. It seems appropriate that the person whose genome was sequenced was James Watson, one of the scientists who received the Nobel Prize in Physiology or Medicine in 1962 for the discovery of the structure of DNA.

Do we have the technology to sequence the genome of cancer cells? The good news is yes we do. We have done it. Using the new sequencing technology called massively parallel sequencing, the three-billion-nucleotide sequence of tumor cells from a woman with acute myeloid leukemia was sequenced and, moreover, was compared to the genomic sequence of some of her healthy cells.

The importance of parallel sequencing of the patient's normal genome is to distinguish tumor-specific mutations from inherited variations. Technology will pave the way to personalized medicine because knowing a particular tumor's molecular defects will allow better choice of treatment for that patient. Research into tumor mutations is being amplified by the work of The Cancer Genome Atlas (TCGA) and the International Cancer Genome Consortium. The latter aims to sequence 500 tumor genomes from 50 of the most common types of cancer and the data will be freely available on the internet.

Companies are also helping to push progress along by offering sequencing services to collaborators in academic, pharmaceutical, and governmental research institutions. Complete Genomics is one such company that will help facilitate the transition of personalized medicine from just an idea to a practical reality. It claims to have the ability to sequence and analyze more than 400 complete human genomes per month, and expects this capacity to increase between two- and three-fold in 2011. Computer giant IBM is in the race and aims to make a nanoscale DNA sequencer on computer-like chips to bring down the cost of sequencing an individual human genome to $1000. Complete individual human tumor genome sequencing will soon become routine in the clinic for the assessment of cancer risk as well as for the choice of treatment. This will call for computerized medical records with large data-storage capabilities. Governments will need to ensure that such information is secure and is not available to be used in harmful ways by employers and insurance companies.

TO THIS, ADD THE COMPLEXITY OF YOUR
INHERITED GENOME

The discussion above focuses on the genetic profile of the tumor but note that this information lies against the background of an individual's inherited genome. This can be thought of as the 'clean slate' that we were born with, our DNA sequence prior to years of exposure to external carcinogens. Variations among individuals define subsets of a population that respond differently to drugs or cancer risk. Some people have genes that cause the build-up of specific drugs and they may be more vulnerable to drug toxicities. These patients will respond better to lower doses of a drug. A specific example is illustrated by the genetic variation in the enzyme thiopurine methyltransferase (TPMT). TPMT-deficient patients accumulate certain chemotherapies, such as 6-mercaptopurine and 6-thioguanine used to treat some leukemias, and this leads to life-threatening toxicity. Successful treatment of these patients can occur with 10–15-fold lower dosage, but there is a need to test patients before treatment and to date such pharmacogenetic tests are not in routine use. Other patients may clear a drug from the body more efficiently due to the nature of their drug-metabolizing enzymes; these patients may have a higher risk of cancer recurrence at a standard drug dose. In the future, the dose of a drug may be able to be adjusted for individual patients based on their genomic information. These few examples underlie the complexity of administering cancer treatments.

Inherited genetic variations are associated with cancer risk. Racial disparities in cancer risk between White people and people of African descent are well documented. Recent evidence suggests that inherited genetic variations contribute to minority disparities in cancer. For instance, Mary Relling and colleagues from the St Jude Children's Research Hospital, Tennessee, reported that an inherited genetic variation (ARID5B) contributes to racial differences in the risk of acute lymphoblastic leukemia. Additional studies that examine genetic variations between ethnic groups and specific cancers are needed.

GENETIC SELECTION AGAINST CANCER FOR THE NEXT GENERATION

Learning about our own personal genome may affect our children. Headline news was made when a woman from a family with three generations of breast cancer screened her IVF embryos for a gene she knew she carried. She eliminated the increased risk of breast cancer that her children would suffer if they were to inherit the gene. At present, only a few germline mutations are known to greatly increase cancer risk in offspring but technology has provided us with new options on how to use this information.

USING *YOUR* CELLS TO TREAT *YOU*

Not long ago it was a fantasy to think that you could boost your own immune cells to fight cancer. This fantasy now a possibility for advanced prostate cancer. Provenge, made by the Dendreon Corporation and approved by the FDA in 2010, is a vaccine made from a patient's immune cells. After removal, cells are activated in the laboratory using a prostate cancer protein and redelivered to the patient in a process that is similar to a blood transfusion. Clinical trials have shown that men treated in this manner lived an average of about four months longer than control patients, who were not treated in this way. Though far from a cure, this approach buys time and hope for some patients. This is an example of a different type of personalized medicine.

GENE THERAPY FOR CANCER

In a sense, gene therapy is another type of personalized medicine. Gene therapy for cancer involves the delivery of a normal or modified gene into cells to treat cancer. Since tumor suppressor genes are often mutated in cancers, one goal is to add a normal copy of the defective tumor suppressor gene. Most commonly, scientists have tapped into the natural talents of viruses that are able to inject their genome into cells, and have used them to carry 'therapeutic' genes into cells. The viruses are altered to try to make them safe for humans, but unfortunately experience has shown that adverse events are still possible. Alternatively, another goal may be to interfere with the expression of an oncogene. A new technology that may be used to accomplish this goal of gene therapy is RNA interference (RNAi). This is an RNA technology that can be used to block the expression of a chosen gene.

Most of the clinical trials in gene therapy performed in 28 countries are carried out with the aim of treating cancer (about 67% of all gene therapy trials). Although gene therapy has not fulfilled our great expectations to date, gene therapy for cancer is on the horizon and even closer if you live in China. China now has two licensed gene therapy agents, Gendicine and H101, which are being used to treat thousands of patients. Gendicine introduces the *p53* gene and its product, P53, is the star player in suppressing tumors. It can trigger DNA repair and even the death of a cell if it contains extensive DNA damage. It can also block blood vessels that supply food and oxygen to a tumor. There are some concerns about the safety and efficiency of the China-approved therapies from researchers in other parts of the world because of a lack of peer-reviewed publications about them. In general, the biggest obstacle for gene therapy has been targeting; that is, getting the therapeutic gene into *all* of the target (tumor) cells. Note that in many other countries gene therapy for cancer is an experimental treatment that is currently only available as part of a clinical trial.

THE GOOD NEWS

As futurist Ray Kurzwell has noted, health medicine and biology are now information technologies. Information technology has not grown in a linear fashion, but rather exponentially, an observation made in 1965 by Gordon Moore, cofounder of Intel, known as Moore's Law. One only needs to think about the computer power available 20 years ago, and compare it to the smart phones of today, to understand the rate of progress that is predicted for the next 20 years. The good news is that the use of an individual's genome and their tumor genome as an information technology promises to yield monumental advances in cancer treatment in the near future. Personalized medicine will pay off. It will lead to better and more effective care in less time, with fewer complications and side-effects, at a lower cost.

14

WHERE DO WE GO FROM HERE?

We are entering a technological dream with cancer. Molecular diagnostics, personalised medicine, precision radiotherapy and targeted logically designed drugs will dramatically improve the quality of life for our patients.

Karol Sikora, Medical Director, CancerPartnersUK

Make no mistakes, cancer is still a hideous disease and accounts of more deaths of people under the age of 85 than any other disease. Initial progress is reported in this book but we still have a long way to go before the disease is conquered.

We must not be complacent, but instead increase our efforts and investments in cancer control. An obvious direction that needs to be taken is to spread good practice. Smoking bans need to be set up in the East, such as China, where lung cancer rates are soaring. Screening and vaccination programs need to be set up in developing countries. In their report prepared for the International Union Against Cancer, Machlin and colleagues (2009) stated that in contrast to Northern and Western Europe, America, and

Australia and New Zealand, where more than two in three people have been screened for cancer, fewer than one in five people have been screened for cancer in Africa and Asia. Consequently, Africans and Asians may be diagnosed at later stages, when outcomes are not as positive. This may partly explain why Africans and Asians are more pessimistic about cures for cancer. Development and dissemination of easier screening methods will not only help diagnose cancer at an earlier stage but also raise hope in these locations. Most importantly, cancer awareness must be raised so that lifestyle changes can be made. It is important to reverse the rising trends in obesity and alcohol consumption in the developed world. Perhaps future genomic technologies will provide the personalized evidence needed for individuals to listen to prevention advice.

An issue that has been flagged for consideration by David Hemenway (2010) is the lack of spending on public health. Public health is involved in disease prevention and early diagnosis and could greatly reduce cancer mortality. But Hemenway believes public health involves forward thinking and does not produce immediate and easily measureable outcomes and so can be neglected by politicians who need to show short-term effectiveness. Public health is different from clinical medicine in that medicine deals with individuals and public health deals with populations of people, measured by statistics. Leaders in public health initiatives are seldom known. Public health policies often face opposition. It is time to invest and embrace public health initiatives.

Cost will be a challenge for the future. Dr Karol Sikora, a leading cancer expert in the UK and advisor to the World Health Organization, summed it up by saying 'the future is going to get more expensive'. Cost-effectiveness of cancer drugs is a controversial topic. The recommendation against the use of Avastin (bevacizumab) for metastatic colon cancer by the UK National Institute for Health and Clinical Excellence (NICE; an advisory agency for the National Health Service), in part because it was deemed not to be a cost-effective use of resources, made headlines and was the topic of debate. Further still, it is estimated that 70% of the global cancer burden in 2020 will be in the developing world. The financial management of this problem will not be easy, noting that in 2008 the National Health Service spent approximately $3,000 per capita in the UK, compared to Kenya where $8.30 per capita was spent on healthcare. Some pharmaceutical companies have made positive contributions to solving the problem by providing free drugs to low-income countries. The Glivec International Patient Assistance Program offered by Novartis is an example of a project that provides such a service in about 80 different countries. It would be beneficial to all if clinical information were collected from treated populations to feed back and enhance the understanding of the drug and refine future treatment schedules. A concerted effort from multiple agencies will be needed to improve cancer care in low-income countries.

CANCER CONCEPTS OF THE FUTURE

Drug combinations

In a talk at the Cleveland Clinic Medical Innovations summit 2009, James Doroshow, Director of Cancer Treatment and Diagnosis at the National Cancer Institute, discussed cancer concepts of the last five years and predicted those of the next five years. Combination targeted therapy (or combination chemotherapy) is one concept on his list that will continue to see growth over the next few years. The use of agents in combination often appears to have improved benefit. For example, significant enhanced clinical activity in multiple myeloma patients is seen with the combination of lenalidomide, bortezomib, and dexamethasone compared to each agent alone. Strategies may include using several drugs aimed at one target for enhanced inhibition (such as two different drugs that target VEGF receptor), drugs aimed at multiple targets with a pathway (EGF receptor and MAPK), or multiple targets in parallel pathways (drugs that target the VEGF receptor and the EGF receptor). The company Zalicus, based in Cambridge, Massachusetts, is a biopharmaceutical company that is using a robotic experimental system that allows the testing of thousands of compounds for synergistic activity (that is, being better than each one alone) when combined. Richard Rickles, Director of Oncology at Zalicus, and colleagues reported a novel synergistic combination targeting two distinct pathways (inhibiting growth and triggering apoptosis) of lymphoma and myeloma cell lines. This suggests that the newly identified combination may have potential clinical value.

Stem cell therapeutics

Stem cell therapeutics is another concept for cancer drug development in the future on Doroshow's list. This topic can be discussed in two very different contexts. The first involves the use of stem cells to help rebuild tissues damaged by cancer and is considered regenerative medicine. The second involves the development of drugs that target the stem cells within a tumor, so-called cancer stem cells.

Stem cells have caused much hype over the last decade, not surprisingly, because they are simply remarkable. We seldom think about how each one of us arose from a single cell, the fertilized egg. The process whereby a complete person containing hundreds of different cell types develops from the fertilized egg and its immediate daughter cells, unspecialized embryonic stem cells, is almost magical. During development the different cell types produced by embryonic stem cells are organized into different tissues, organs, and patterns. In addition to the stem cells of the embryo, there are also stem cells in the adult that help regenerate tissues over the lifetime of an individual. Some of these stem cells work continuously to replace cells as they die off, such as the skin. Others respond to physiological signals: breast stem cells respond to pregnancy hormones causing breasts to nearly double in size during pregnancy, and hair follicle stem cells respond to a wound. The defining characteristics of a stem cell are that it can both self-renew, forming more stem cells, and also give rise to more specialized cell types. Thus blood stem cells produce additional blood stem cells and also give rise to all of the specialized cells of the blood (e.g. white blood cells and red blood cells). Adult stem cells do not demonstrate the ability to form *all* of the cell types in the body like embryonic stem cells and so are more limited in their application. In addition to these two types of stem cells, we can create cells similar to embryonic stem cells from adult cells, called induced pluripotent cells, in the laboratory. Over the last decade scientists have learned ways of harvesting and directing the specialization of stem cells and are trying to apply this knowledge to clinical applications.

The idea that stem cell therapy may be used to replace tissue damaged by cancer sounds futuristic, but in fact has been carried out for decades in leukemia patients. A bone marrow transplant, where the bone marrow of a matched donor is transplanted into a leukemia patient to restore the blood system of the patient whose marrow has been irradiated to kill leukemic cells, is a stem cell therapy. Further progress with stem cells is underway. The demonstration of a successful tracheal transplant in a 30-year-old woman with tuberculosis opened the door for similar work to be carried out for cancer patients. The tracheal transplant involved using a donor trachea from a cadaver (after removing donor cells and antigens), seeding it with cells grown in the laboratory from the patient's own stem cells, and surgically replacing the patient's diseased trachea (Macchiarini et al., 2008). The patient did not require immunosuppressive drugs and had a functional airway immediately and up to four months after surgery, the time the report was written. This procedure has been repeated by Paulo Macchiarini and colleagues for two women of 31 and 19 years with a primary tracheal malignant cancer not amenable to standard therapy and both transplantations went well (P. Macchiarini, personal communication). Bioartificial organs made from stem cells and artificial scaffolds are being developed to treat cancer damage, such as liver failure. Stem cell medicine promises to make significant contributions to future cancer treatments.

The hypothesis that tumor initiation and progression is due to a rare population of stem-like cells was first proposed by John Dick, a Canadian scientist, in the 1990s. These rare stem cell-like cells, called cancer stem cells, were first identified in leukemias, but were also found for many solid cancers. Cancer stem cells are known to be relatively resistant to chemotherapies and radiation and may help explain why many cancers relapse after treatment. In the past we have often measured the effectiveness of a cancer drug by tumor shrinkage. But, if a drug kills the majority of a tumor but fails to kill the rare tumor-initiating cancer stem cells then one can begin to understand why a cancer returns. Future cancer drug development aimed at targeting cancer stem cells may prevent reoccurrence and actually cure metastatic cancer. Several molecular signaling pathways—such as Wnt, Hedgehog, and Notch—demonstrated to be important in stem cell renewal during development are also important in cancer stem cell renewal. Agents that inhibit these pathways are being tested in clinical trials and show promise (Von Hoff et al., 2009). Advances are being made to grow large amounts of cancer stems cells in the laboratory and design cancer stem cell-based assays as tools for finding new drugs that specifically target cancer stem cells.

CANCER PATIENTS AND FERTILITY

In the past, young female cancer patients sacrificed their fertility for survival. This is all set to change with new reproductive technologies. In June 2010, a healthy baby was delivered by the first cancer patient to receive an ovary transplant from frozen tissue obtained before she was treated for cancer. The woman was diagnosed with Hodgkin lymphoma at the age of 19 and before she was treated for her cancer she had her ovarian tissue frozen. Ovarian transplantation from frozen tissue was carried out 13 years later after several cancer reoccurrences, multiple rounds of chemotherapy and radiotherapy, and two bone marrow transplants, procedures that leave patients sterile. The procedure, carried out at The Infertility

Center of St Louis, Missouri, by Dr Sherman Silber and colleagues, is now considered robust and easy to carry out. The eggs of the ovary are housed in the rim of the organ. This tissue can be surgically removed in a one-hour procedure and frozen for future transplantation. Similar to a skin graft, pieces of the outer rim of the ovary can be transplanted onto the surface of an ovary with several sutures. Soon after, the ovary functions as usual, monthly cycles are resumed, and women can become pregnant without any additional medical interventions. At the Medical Innovations Summit of the Royal Society of Medicine in 2010 Dr Silber retold the surprising reaction of the 31-year-old cancer survivor: she said, 'You know, I feel so fortunate that I had cancer. My girlfriends in their 30s are all worried about their biological clock, but I have a 19-year-old ovary and I am, ironically, even more fertile than they are.'

The procedure was originally carried out on female identical twins where one of the twins was infertile. Identical twins arise when one early embryo splits into two. If the splitting occurs later rather than earlier, cells that produce eggs remain in one twin and are absent in the other. Dr Silber has extended this procedure to help cancer patients.

NEW TECHNOLOGIES CHANGE THE WAY
WE TREAT CANCER

New technologies change the way we do things in all aspects of life and they will continue to drive progress in cancer management. A search using 'cancer' as a keyword in a UK database of British technology companies, called the Gibson Index (www.Gibson-index. com), yielded more than 250 companies. The profiles of companies indicated their involvement in diverse activities including specialist software applications, imaging, detection of carcinogens, diagnosis, patient care, and drug screening. One company featured in the search is Ambicare Health. They developed a technology called Ambulight PDT (which stands for photodynamic therapy), a light-emitting band aid or plaster for the treatment of non-melanoma skin cancer that transforms a patient's treatment experience. Photodynamic therapy is a well-established alternative to surgery for some skin cancers. It involves the application of a pharmaceutical that becomes active in the presence of a light source to kill cancer cells. In contrast to conventional PDT, the Ambulight PDT, once fitted by a heathcare professional, allows independence from a hospital setting, reduces overhead hospital costs, and allows the patient to move around their own home. The CE-marked medical device was launched in Europe in late 2009.

Surgery has been the primary means of cancer treatment. Its precision has greatly improved over recent times. But what if surgery is not an option? A new field of radiology, called interventional radiology, based on new technologies, uses minimally invasive procedures guided by imaging techniques such as ultrasound, magnetic resonance imaging (MRI), and computed tomography (CT) (note: CT uses ionizing radiation and therefore must be used conservatively) (Katsanos et al., 2009). Many people may be aware of the technique called angioplasty, a type of interventional radiology, used in cardiac medicine. For cancer, examples of interventional radiology are radiofrequency ablation and high-intensity focused ultrasound (HIFU). HIFU has been used to treat prostate cancer and more recently it has been trialed to treat colon cancer in an 88-year-old patient who was not a candidate for surgery.

A transducer is inserted into the colon and is used to focus an ultra-sound wave, similar to the focusing of sunlight by a magnifying glass. This thermal therapy can heat targeted tissue up to 80–90 degrees Celsius and kill tumor cells. The procedure was reported to have immediately increased the quality of life for the patient. The Cyberknife, manufactured by Accuray Inc., uses a high dose of radiation to ablate a tumor as an alternative to surgery. This procedure is referred to as radiosurgery and uses real-time imaging to guide a robotics system. Positive outcomes have been reported for lung and prostate cancer but time is needed to examine long-term effects. Advances in imaging technology such as the new Magnetom Skyra 3 Tesla MRI System by Siemens (see Figure 21

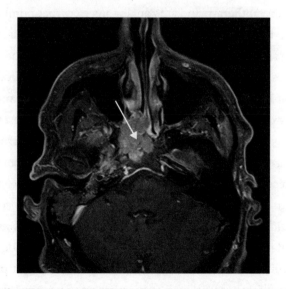

FIG 21 MRI image using the Magnetom Skyra 3 Tesla MRI System by Siemens. A tumor is indicated by the arrow.

for a representative image) allows us to see and understand cancer better. Improved imaging systems, including molecular-functional imaging that examines molecular pathways and tissue function, will continue to make large contributions to cancer management in the future.

Nanomedicine as a means of drug delivery to targeted cells is another area that promises to deliver better cancer treatments soon. By definition, these agents are tiny, having one dimension in the 1–1000 nanometer range (1000 nanometers = 0.001 millimeters). For reference this means they range from the size of a few atoms to the size of structures inside of a cell. The power of targeting a lethal drug specifically to cancer cells is analogous to the power of guided missiles in military conflicts. As described in an editorial by P.A. McCarron and A.M. Faheem, the administration of chemotherapy today is analogous to carpet bombing and the time has come to commission the therapeutic cruise missile (McCarron and Faheem, 2010). The current design of such a therapeutic is a drug-filled particle with a molecular tag on the outside that can deliver it to the molecular address of a cancer cell. In many cases the tag is like the key-and-lock model described in Chapter 5 for a growth factor and its receptor. Transferrin is one molecular tag being used to target the increased number of transferrin receptors on metastatic and drug-resistant cells. Nanoparticles can also be made magnetic by use of iron oxide to construct the particle. Such particles can be guided by an applied magnetic field and monitored by MRI. Nanotechnology will also be applied to make biomolecular sensors that will be able to detect many biochemical molecules (known as biomarkers) for refined diagnosis and treatment monitoring. One design, called the nanocantilever, resembles a piano keyboard and moves like a tapped key when it binds to a biomarker. These small movements are monitored by lasers. It is hoped that such technology will replace the need for biopsies.

TEAMWORK

Progress in cancer management takes teamwork. Both drug development and clinical management involve expertise in many disciplines. We have begun to witness the creation of extremely powerful teams; teams that not only cross academic institutional departments, but teams that unite different academic institutions with each other and with biotechnology and pharmaceutical companies. There are teams that share state-of-the-art facilities across different medical centers and teams that transcend international borders. Patients are becoming a bigger part of the team. Pharmaceutical giants are tremendous teams in themselves that serve as a crucial link in bringing basic science to the bedside. They are *the* producers of the new molecular targeted cancer drugs such Avastin (made by Genentech), Gleevec (Novartis), Iressa (AstraZeneca), Nexavar (Bayer), Sutent (Pfizer), Tykerb (GlaxoSmithKline), and Zolinza (Merck). A faster rate of progress and better care is an obvious outcome of teamwork.

THE GOOD NEWS

We, as a team, can now build on our early successes. The good news is that we are seeing the beginning of the end.

BIBLIOGRAPHY

Chapter 1

DiMasi, J.A., Feldman, L., Seckler, A., and Wilson, A. (2010) Trends in risks associated with new drug development: success rates for investigational new drugs. *Clinical Pharmacology and Therapeutics* 87:272–277.

Jemal, A., Siegal, R., Xu, J., and Ward, E. (2010a) Cancer Statistics, 2010. *CA: a Cancer Journal for Clinicians* 60:277–300.

Jemal, A., Ward, E., and Thun, M. (2010b) Declining death rates reflect progress against cancer. *PLoS ONE* 5 (3):e9584.

Kaatsch, P. (2010) Epidemiology of childhood cancer. *Cancer Treatment Reviews* 36:277–285.

Machlin, A., Wakefield, M., Spittal, M., and Hill, D. (2009) *Cancer-related Beliefs and Behaviours in Eight Geographical Regions.* Prepared for the International Union Against Cancer. January 2009. www. uicc.org/sites/clonesource.agenceinovae.com/files/survey%20 report.pdf.

National Cancer Institute (2010) *Cancer Trends Progress Report— 2009/2010 Update.* April 2010. http://progressreport.cancer.gov.

Stephens, P.J., Greenman, C.D., Fu, B., Yang, F., Bignell, G.R., Mudie, L.J., Pleasance, E.D., Lau, K.W., Beare, D., Stebbings, L.A. et al. (2011) Massive genomic rearrangement acquired in a single catastrophic event during cancer development. *Cell* 144:27–40.

Chapter 2

Citron, M.L., Berry, D.A., Cirrincione, C., Hudis, C., Winer, E.P., Gradishar, W.J., Davidson, N.E., Martino, S., Livingston, R., Ingle, J.N. et al. (2003) Randomized trial of dose-dense versus conventionally scheduled and sequential versus concurrent combination chemotherapy as postoperative adjuvant treatment of node-positive primary breast cancer: first report of Intergroup Trial C9741/Cancer and Leukemia Group B Trial 9741. *Journal of Clinical Oncology* 21:1431–1439.

Dulbecco, R. (1986) A turning point in cancer research: sequencing the human genome. *Science* 7:1055–1056.

Futreal, P.A., Colin, L., Marshall, M., Down, T., Hubbard, T., Wooster, R., Rahman, N., and Stratton, M.R. (2004) A census of human cancer genes. *Nature Reviews Cancer* 4:117–183.

Gibbs, W.W. (2008) Untangling the roots of cancer. *Scientific American* 18:30–39.

Hanahan, D. and Weinberg, R.A. (2011) Hallmarks of cancer: the next generation. *Cell* 144:646–674.

Martling, A.L., Holm, T., Rutqvist, L.-E., Moran, B.J., Heald, R.J., and Cedermark, B. (2000) Effect of a surgical training programme on outcome of rectal cancer in the county of Stockholm. *The Lancet* 356:93–96.

Chapter 3

Beral, V. and Million Woman Study Collaborators (2003) Breast cancer and hormone replacement therapy in the Million Woman Study. *The Lancet* 362:419–427.

Ghanei, M. and Harandi, A.A. (2010) Lung carcinogenicity of sulfur mustard. *Clinical Lung Cancer* 11:13–17.

Gundestrup, M. and Storm, H.H. (1999) Radiation-induced acute myeloid leukemia and other cancers in commercial jet cockpit crew: a population-based cohort study. *The Lancet* 354:2029–2031.

Little, M.P. (2009) Cancer and non-cancer effects in Japanese atomic bomb survivors. *Journal of Radiological Protection* 29: A43.

National Cancer Institute (2003) *Cancer and the Environment: What You Need to Know, What You Can Do.* U.S. Department of Health and Human Services. August 2003. www.cancer.gov/images/Documents/5d17e03e-b39f-4b40-a214-e9e9099c4220/Cancer%20and%20the%20Environment.pdf.

Preston, D.L., Shimizu, Y., Pierce, D.A., Suyama, A., and Mabuchi, K. (2003) Studies of mortality of atomic bomb survivors. Report 13: solid cancer and noncancer disease mortality; 1950–1997. *Radiation Research* 160:381–407.

Seitz, H.K. and Stickel, F. (2007) Molecular mechanisms of alcohol-mediated carcinogenesis. *Nature Reviews Cancer* 7:599–612.

Chapter 4

Aldington, S., Harwood, M., Cox, B., Weatherall, M., Beckert, L., Hansell, A., Pritchard, A., Robinson, G., and Beasley, R., Cannabis and Respiratory Disease Research Group (2008) Cannabis use and risk of lung cancer: a case-control study. *European Respiratory Journal* 31:280–286.

BBC News (2009) China orders officials to smoke. May 2009. http://news.bbc.co.uk/go/pr/fr/-/1/hi/world/asia-pacific/8033101.stm.

Cassidy, A., Myles, J.P., Duffy, S.W., Liloglou, T., and Field, J.K. (2006) Family history and risk of lung cancer: age-at-diagnosis in cases and first-degree relatives. *British Journal of Cancer* 95:1288–1290.

Chanock, S.J. and Hunter, D.J. (2008) When the smoke clears....*Nature* 452:537–539.

Darby, S., Hill, D., Auvinen, A., Barros-Dios, J.M., Baysson, H., Bochicchio, F., Deo, H., Falk, R., Forastiere, F., Hakama, M. et al. (2005) Radon in homes and risk of lung cancer: collaborative analysis of individual data from 13 European case-control studies. *British Medical Journal* 330:223–228.

Denissenko, M.F., Pao, A., Tang, M.-S., and Pfeifer, G.P. (1996) Preferential formation of benzo[a]pyrene adducts at lung cancer mutational hotspots in *p53*. *Science* 274:430–432.

Deyton, L., Sharfstein, J., and Hamburg, M. (2010) Tobacco product regulation—a public health approach. *New England Journal of Medicine* 362:1753–1756.

Doll, R. and Hill, B. (1954) The mortality of doctors in relation to their smoking habits: a preliminary report. Reprinted: *British Medical Journal* (2004) 328:1529–1533.

Doll, R., Peto, R., Boreham, J., and Sutherland, I. (2004) Mortality in relation to smoking: 50 years' observations on male British doctors. *British Medical Journal* 328:1519–1528.

Dubey, S. and Powell, C.A. (2008) Update in Lung Cancer 2007. *American Journal of Respiratory and Critical Care Medicine* 177:941–946.

Gruer, L., Hart, C.L., Gordon, D.S., and Watt, G.C.M. (2009) Effect of tobacco smoking on survival of men and woman by social position: a 28 year cohort study. *British Medical Journal* 338:b480.

Gu, D., Kelly, T.N., Wu, X., Chen, J., Samet, J.M., Huang, J.-F., Zhu, M., Chen, J.-C., Chen, C.-S., Duan, X. et al. (2009) Mortality attributable to smoking in China. *New England Journal of Medicine* 360:150–159.

IARC (2009) *IARC Handbooks of Cancer Prevention: Tobacco Control. Vol. 13. Evaluating the Effectiveness of Smoke-free Policies.* International Agency for Research on Cancer, Lyon.

McKay, J.D., Hung, R.J., Gaborieau, V., Boffetta, P., Chabrier, A., Byrnes, G., Zaridze, D., Mukeria, A., Szeszenia-Dabrowska, N., Lissowska, J. et al. (2008) Lung cancer susceptibility locus at 5p15.33. *Nature Genetics* 40:1404–1406.

Peto, R., Darby, S., Deo, H., Silcocks, P., Whitley, E., and Doll, R. (2000) Smoking, smoking cessation, and lung cancer in the UK since 1950: combination of national statistics with two-case-control studies. *British Medical Journal* 321:323–329.

Smith, C.J., Perfetti, T.A., Garg, R., and Hansch, C. (2003) IARC carcinogens reported in cigarette mainstream smoke and their calculated log P values. *Food and Chemical Toxicology* 41:807–817.

Wynder, E.L. and Graham, E. (1950) Tobacco smoking as a possible etiologic factor in bronchiogenic carcinoma: a study of 684 proven cases. *Journal of the American Medical Association* 143:329–336.

Map of radon zones in the USA. http://www.epa.gov/radon/pdfs/zonemapcolor.pdf

Map of radon affected areas in the UK. http://www.ukradon.org/article.php?key=indicativemap_EW

Chapter 5

Krause, D.S. and Van Etten, R.A. (2005) Tyrosine kinases as targets for cancer therapy. *New England Journal of Medicine* 353:172–187.

Pecorino, L. (2008) Growth factor signaling and oncogenes. In *The Molecular Biology of Cancer: Mechanisms, Targets, and Therapeutics*, 2nd edn, pp. 69–94. Oxford University Press, Oxford.

Stix, G. (2006) Blockbuster dreams. *Scientific American* 294:60–63.

Chapter 6

Christofori, G. (2006) New signals from the invasive front. *Nature* 441:444–450.

Fidler, I.J. and Langley, R.R. (2007) Tumor cell-organ microenvironment interactions in the pathogenesis of cancer metastasis. *Endocrine Reviews* 28:297–321.

Geiger, T.R. and Peeper, D.S. (2009) Metastasis mechanisms. *Biochemica et Biophysical Acta* 1796:293–308.

Hunter, K.W. (2004) Host genetics and tumor metastasis. *British Journal of Cancer* 90:752–755.

Kaplan, R.N., Shahin, R., and Lyden, D. (2006) Preparing the 'soil': the premetastatic niche. *Cancer Research* 66:11089–11093.

Minn, A.J., Gupta, G.P., Siegel, P.M., Bos, P.D., Shu, W., Giri, D.D., Viale, A., Olshen, A.B., Gerald, W.L., and Massagué, J. (2005) Genes that mediate breast cancer metastasis to the lung. *Nature* 436:518–524.

Nguyen, D.X., Bos, P.D., and Massagué, J. (2009) Metastasis: from dissemination to organ-specific colonization. *Nature Reviews Cancer* 9:274–284.

Wyckoff, J.B., Wang, Y., Lin, E.Y., Li, J.-F., Goswami, S., Stanley, E.R., Segall, J.E., Pollard, J.W., and Condeelis, J. (2007) Direct visualization of macrophage-assisted tumor cell intravasation in mammary tumors. *Cancer Research* 67:2649–2656.

Chapter 7

Coghlan, A. (2010) Cancer's sweet tooth becomes a target. *New Scientist* 2760:12 May.

Key, T.J., Allen, N.E., Spencer, E.A., and Travis, R.C. (2002) The effect of diet on risk of cancer. *The Lancet* 360:861–868.

World Cancer Research Fund/American Institute for Cancer Research (2007) *Food, Nutrition, Physical Activity, and the Prevention of Cancer: a Global Perspective.* American Institute for Cancer Research, Washington DC. www.dietandcancerreport.org/.

World Cancer Research Fund/American Institute for Cancer Research (2009) *Policy and Action for Cancer Prevention.* American Institute for Cancer Research, Washington DC.

Chapter 8

Daley, G.Q., Van Etten, R.A., and Baltimore, D. (1990) Induction of chronic myelogenous leukemia in mice by the P210*bcr/abl* gene of the Philadelphia chromosome. *Science* 247:824–830.

Druker, B.J. (2008) Translation of the Philadelphia chromosome into therapy for CML. *Blood* 112:4808–4817.

Martindale, D. (2001) Cancer in the crosshairs: why some tumors withstand Gleevec's Targeted Assault. *Scientific American* 285:19–20.

Chapter 9

American Cancer Society. *American Cancer Society Guidelines for the Early Detection of Cancer.* www.cancer.org/docroot/PED/content/PED_2_3X_ACS_Cancer_Detection_Guidelines_36.asp?sitearea=PED.

Boyle, P., Autier, P., Bartelink, H., Baselga, J., Boffetta, P., Burn, J., Burns, H.J., Christensen, L., Denis, L., Dicato, M. et al. (2003) European Code against Cancer and scientific justification: third version. *Annals of Oncology* 14:973–1005.

Cancer Research UK (2009) *Screening and Cancer: the Evidence.* September 2009. http://info.cancerresearchuk.org/spotcancerearly/screening/evidenceforscreening/.

Department of Health and Aging, Australian Government. Homepage. www.cancerscreening.gov.au/.

Gøtzsche, P.C. and Nielsen, M. (2011) Screening for breast cancer with mammography. *Cochrane Database of Systematic Reviews* 1:CD001877.

Imperiale, T.F., Ransohoff, D.F., Itzkowitz, S.H., Turnbull, B.A., and Ross, M.E. (2004) Fecal DNA versus fecal occult blood for colorectal-cancer screening in an average-risk population. *New England Journal of Medicine* 351:2704–2714.

International Agency for Research on Cancer (2002) Mammography screening can reduce deaths from breast cancer. Press release 39. March 2002. www.iarc.fr/en/media-centre/pr/2002/pr139.html.

Itzkowitz, S., Brand, R., Jandorf, L., Durkee, K., Millholland, J., Rabeneck, L., Schroy 3rd, P.C., Sontag, S., Johnson, D., Markowitz, S. et al. (2008) A simplified, noninvasive stool DNA test for colorectal cancer detection. *American Journal of Gastroenterology* 103:2862–2870.

National Cancer Information Fact Sheet. *Prostate Specific Antigen (PSA) Test.* www.cancer.gov/cancertopics/factsheet/Detection/PSA.

National Cancer Institute, The Early Detection Research Network (2008) *Investing in Translational Research on Biomarkers of Early Cancer and Cancer Risk*, fourth report. http://edrn.nci.nih.gov/docs/progress-reports/edrn_4th-report_200801.pdf.

Smith, R.A., Cokkinides, V., and Brawley, O.W. (2009) Cancer screening in the United States, 2009. *CA: a Cancer Journal for Clinicians* 59:27–41.

Chapter 10

Bailey, D.S. and Zanders, E.D. (2008) Drug discovery in the era of Facebook—new tools for scientific networking. *Drug Discovery Today* 13:863–868.

Morra, M.E., Van Nevel, J.P., Nealon, E.O'D., Mazan, K.D., and Thomsen, C. (1993) History of the Cancer Information Service. *Journal of the National Cancer Institute Monographs* 14:7–33.

Viswanath, K., Herbst, R.S., Land, S.R., Leischow, S.J., and Shields, P.G. (2010) Tobacco and cancer: an American Association for Cancer Research Policy Statement. *Cancer Research* 70:3420–3430.

Chapter 11

Cao, Y. and Langer, R. (2008) A review of Judah Folkman's remarkable achievements in biomedicine. *Proceedings of the National Academy of Sciences USA* 105:13203–13205.

Ferrara, N., Hillan, K.J., Gerber, H.-P., and Novotny, W. (2004) Discovery and development of Bevacizumab, an anti-VEGF antibody for treating cancer. *Nature Reviews Drug Discovery* 3:391–400.

Folkman, J. (1971) Tumor angiogenesis: therapeutic implications. *New England Journal of Medicine* 285:1182–1186.

Knies-Bamforth, U. and Watson, C. (2005) Napoleone Ferrara discusses Avastin and the future of anti-angiogenesis therapy. *Drug Discovery Today* 10:539–541.

Chapter 12

American Society of Cancer. *Human Papilloma Virus (HPV), Cancer, and HPV Vaccines—Frequently Asked Questions.* www.cancer. org/docroot/CRI/content/CRI_2_6x_FAQ_HPV_Vaccines. asp?sitearea=.

Cancer Research UK. *HPV Vaccines.* www.cancerhelp.org.uk/about-cancer/cancer-questions/cervical-cancer-vaccine.

Centers for Disease Control and Prevention. *Sexually Transmitted Diseases: Genital HPV Infection Fact Sheet.* www.cdc.gov/STD/HPV/ STDFact-HPV.htm.

Centers for Disease Control and Prevention. *Vaccines and Immunizations: HPV Vaccine: Questions and Answers.* www.cdc.gov/vaccines/ vpd-vac/hpv/vac-faqs.htm.

Fenner, F., Anderson, D., Arita, I., Jezek, Z., and Ladnyi, I. (1988) *Smallpox and Its Eradication.* World Health Organization, Geneva.

Lowy, D.R. and Schiller, J.T. (2006) Prophylactic human papillomavirus vaccines. *Journal of Clinical Investigation* 116:1167–1173.

Riedel, S. (2005) Edward Jenner and the history of smallpox and vaccination. *Proceedings (Baylor University Medical Center)* 18:21–25.

Stewart, A.J. and Devlin, P.M. (2006) The history of the smallpox vaccine. *Journal of Infection* 52:329–334.

Chapter 13

Fong, P.C., Boss, D.S., Yap, T.A., Tutt, A., Wu, P., Mergui-Roelvink, M., Mortimer, P., Swaisland, H., Lau, A., O'Connor, M.J. et al. (2009) Inhibition of poly (AD-Ribose) polymerase in tumors from BRCA mutation carriers. *New England Journal of Medicine* 361:123–134.

Ley, T.J., Mardis, E.R., Ding, L., Fulton, B., McLellan, M.D., Chen, K., Dooling, D., Dunford-Shore, B.H., McGrath, S., Hickenbotham, M. et al. (2008) DNA sequencing of a cytogenetically normal acute myeloid leukemia genome. *Nature* 456:66–72.

Malone, B. (2010) NCI launches national biobank. *American Association of Clinical Chemistry* 36:1–7.

National Cancer Institute. *Fact Sheet TAILORx*. www.cancer.gov/cancertopics/factsheet/therapy/tailorx.

National Cancer Institute. *NCI Fact Sheet. Gene Therapy for Cancer: Questions and Answers*. www.cancer.gov/cancertopics/factsheet/Therapy/gene.

National Comprehensive Cancer Network (2008) *News NCCN Updates Breast Cancer Guidelines*. January 2008. www.nccn.org/about/news/newsinfo.asp?NewsID=127.

Park, A. (2009) 10 ideas changing the world right now. *Times Magazine*, March 12. www.time.com/time/specials/packages/article/0,28804,1884779_1884782_1884766,00.html.

Wheeler, D.A. (2008) The complete genome of an individual by massively parallel DNA sequencing. *Nature* 452:872–877.

Yang, W., Trevino, L.R., Yang, J.J., Scheet, P., Pui, C.H., Evans, W.E., and Relling, M.V. (2010) ARID5B SNP rs10821936 is associated with risk of childhood acute lymphoblastic leukemia in blacks and contributes to racial differences in leukemia incidence. *Leukemia* 24:894–896.

Chapter 14

Hemenway, D. (2010) Why we don't spend enough on public health. *New England Journal of Medicine* 362:1657–1658.

Katsanos, K., Ahmad, F., Dourado, R., Sabharwal, T., and Adam, A. (2009) Interventional radiology in the elderly. *Clinical Interventions in Aging* 4:1–15.

Kerr, D.J. and Midgley, R. (2010) Can we treat cancer for a dollar a day? Guidelines for low-income countries. *New England Journal of Medicine* 363:801–803.

Lee, S.J., Schover, L.R., Partridge, A.H., Patrizio, P., Wallace, W.H., Hagerty, K., Beck, L.N., Brennan, L.V., and Oktay, K. (2006) American Society of Clinical Oncology recommendations on fertility preservation in cancer patients. *Journal of Clinical Oncology* 24:2917–2931.

Macchiarini, P., Jungebluth, P., Go, T., Asnaghi, M.A., Rees, L.E., Cogan, T.A., Dodson, A., Martorell, J., Bellini, S., Parnigotto, P.P. et al. (2008) Clinical transplantation of a tissue-engineered airway. *The Lancet* 372:2023–2030.

Machlin, A., Wakefield, M., Spittal, M., and Hill, D. (2009) *Cancer-related Beliefs and Behaviours in Eight Geographical Regions.* Prepared for the International Union Against Cancer. January 2009. www.uicc.org/sites/clonesource.agenceinovae.com/files/survey%20report.pdf.

McCarron, P.A. and Faheem, A.M. (2010) Nanomedicine-based cancer targeting: a new weapon in an old war. *Nanomedicine* 5:3–5.

Rickles, R.J., Pierce, L.T., Giordano 3rd, T.P., Tam, W., McMillin, D.W., Delmore, J., Laubach, J.P., Borisy, A.A., Richardson, P.G., and Lee, M.S. (2010) Adenosine A2A receptor agonists and PDE inhibitors: a synergistic multitarget mechanism discovered through systematic combination screening in B-cell malignancies. *Blood* 116:593–602.

Silber, S., Kagawa, N., Kuwayama, M., and Gosden, R. (2010) Duration of fertility after fresh and frozen ovary transplantation. *Fertility and Sterility* 94:2191–2196.

Von Hoff, D.D., LoRusso, P.M., Rudin, C.M., Reddy, J.C., Yauch, R.L., Tibes, R., Weiss, G.J., Borad, M.J., Hann, C.L., Brahmer, J.R. et al. (2009) Inhibition of the hedgehog pathway in advanced basal-cell carcinoma. *New England Journal of Medicine* 361:1164–1172.

GLOSSARY

ADJUVANT   A substance that is added to a vaccine to increase the body's immune response.

ALLELE   One form of a specific gene pair, remembering that we have two copies of (almost) every gene. For example, a person may have one brown allele and one blue allele for eye color. One allele may be dominant over the other and in this example brown is dominant over blue. This person will have brown eyes.

ANGIOGENESIS   The formation of new blood vessels from preexisting blood vessels.

BIOBANK   A collection of human biological tissue and associated health information that can be used as a resource for current and future research. Participation in biobanks is important for research that will benefit future generations.

BIOMARKER   A biological molecule found in bodily fluids or tissue that indicates health or disease or the effect of treatment.

CARCINOGEN   An agent that causes cancer.

DNA   (deoxyribonucleic acid) The genetic material of most living things that carries the chemical instructions for the synthesis of proteins. The structure of DNA is a double helix, which is important for the process of DNA replication.

DNA ADDUCT A chemical mask on DNA; the addition of a chemical group to DNA.

GENE A section of DNA sequence that carries the chemical instructions to code for a protein. Proteins are needed for the structure and function of cells over a lifetime. There are about 25,000 genes in the human genome.

GENOME The complete set of genes of an individual or species.

GERMLINE MUTATION A mutation in either egg- or sperm-cell DNA (as opposed to a somatic mutation). Only mutations in germ cells can be passed on to the next generation.

INCIDENCE RATE The number of new cases of cancer (or other disease) in a defined population over a defined period of time.

ION A molecule with a positive or negative charge. They may be created by ionizing radiation and can damage DNA, leading to mutations and cancer.

KINASE An enzyme that adds phosphate groups to proteins. The addition of a phosphate can regulate protein activity, turning it on or off. Kinases are important drug targets.

METASTASIS The spread of cancer cells from a primary tumor to distant sites in the body.

METASTASIS SUPPRESSOR GENE A gene that inhibits any of the steps involved in the spread of cancer cells from a primary tumor to a distant site in the body. Over 20 of such genes have been identified.

MONOCLONAL ANTIBODY A molecule of the immune system that is produced in response to exposure to a foreign body. They can be also be designed and prepared in the laboratory and used as a research tool or therapeutic agent. Herceptin is an example of a therapeutic monoclonal antibody.

MUTATION   A permanent change in the DNA sequence. For example, the replacement of 'A' in the genetic code by a 'C'.

ONCOGENE   A mutated gene that can produce a 'faulty' protein product that contributes to cancer (think oncology).

PHARMACOGENOMICS   The study of the influence of genetic variation on drug response.

PHOSPHORYLATION   The addition of a chemical group, called a phosphate, to a protein. The addition causes a change in shape of a protein and, in doing so, can switch the activity of a protein either on or off. This is an important mechanism of the regulation of proteins.

PREMETASTIC NICHE   A site of future metastasis prepared by host cells upon receiving a signal from the primary tumor prior to the arrival of the metastasizing cell.

PRIMARY TUMOR   The original site of a cancer that can give rise to metastasis upon progression.

PROGNOSIS   The predicted outcome of having a disease.

REACTIVE OXYGEN SPECIES   (ROS) Highly reactive oxygen molecules. They can be produced during normal metabolism that uses oxygen or by the interaction of ionizing radiation with water. They can oxidize DNA and cause mutations that may lead to cancer.

RNA   (ribonucleic acid) The genetic material in some viruses. Also, messenger RNA (mRNA) carries the genetic code transcribed from DNA to the ribosomes for protein synthesis.

Other types of RNA in cells are ribosomal RNA, located in ribosomes, and transfer RNA, which plays an important role in protein synthesis.

SOMATIC MUTATION A mutation in any cell other than a germ cell (i.e. an egg or sperm cell). Mutations in somatic cells cannot be passed on to the next generation.

TERATOGEN An agent that causes birth defects.

TRANSCRIPTION FACTOR A protein that binds to the controlling region of genes and which can regulate gene expression (i.e. turn a gene on or off).

TUMOR SUPPRESSOR GENE A gene with a protein product that plays a role in preventing cancer. Loss of function of these genes by mutation or modification contributes to cancer. Functions of tumor suppressor proteins may include regulation of antioxidant enzymes, cell suicide, or DNA repair, or pausing cell division.

VARIOLATION The practice of introducing smallpox virus to non-immune individuals. The procedure involved using a lancet applied with material from a lesion of a smallpox patient. Although not without risks, immunity against future smallpox exposure was often observed.

INDEX